PSYCHOLOGY PRACTITIONER GUIDEBOOKS

EDITORS
Arnold P. Goldstein, Syracuse University
Leonard Krasner, Stanford University & SUNY at Stony Brook
Sol L. Garfield, Washington University in St. Louis

DRUG THERAPY FOR BEHAVIOR DISORDERS

Pergamon Titles of Related Interest

Belar/Deardorff/Kelly THE PRACTICE OF CLINICAL
HEALTH PSYCHOLOGY

Blanchard/Martin/Dubbert NON-DRUG TREATMENTS FOR
ESSENTIAL HYPERTENSION

Blechman/Brownell HANDBOOK OF BEHAVIORAL MEDICINE
FOR WOMEN

LeBow ADULT OBESITY THERAPY

Russell STRESS MANAGEMENT FOR CHRONIC DISEASE

Thompson BODY IMAGE DISTURBANCE: Assessment
and Treatment

Tunks/Bellissimo BEHAVIORAL MEDICINE:
Concepts and Procedures

Williamson ASSESSMENT OF EATING DISORDERS: Obesity,
Anorexia and Bulimia Nervosa

Winett/King/Altman HEALTH PSYCHOLOGY AND PUBLIC
HEALTH: An Integrative Approach

Related Journals
(Free sample copies available upon request)

ADVANCES IN BEHAVIOUR RESEARCH AND THERAPY
BEHAVIORAL ASSESSMENT
BEHAVIOUR RESEARCH AND THERAPY
CLINICAL PSYCHOLOGY REVIEW
JOURNAL OF BEHAVIOR THERAPY AND
   EXPERIMENTAL PSYCHIATRY
SOCIAL SCIENCES AND MEDICINE

DRUG THERAPY FOR BEHAVIOR DISORDERS
An Introduction

ALAN POLING
Western Michigan University

KENNETH D. GADOW
State University of New York at Stony Brook

JAMES CLEARY
University of Minnesota, Minneapolis
and
Veterans Administration Medical Center, Minneapolis

PERGAMON PRESS
Member of Maxwell Macmillan Pergamon Publishing Corporation
New York • Oxford • Beijing • Frankfurt
São Paulo • Sydney • Tokyo • Toronto

Pergamon Press Offices:

U.S.A.	Pergamon Press, Inc., Maxwell House, Fairview Park, Elmsford, New York 10523, U.S.A.
U.K.	Pergamon Press plc, Headington Hill Hall, Oxford OX3 0BW, England
PEOPLE'S REPUBLIC OF CHINA	Pergamon Press, 0909 China World Tower, No. 1 Jian Guo Men Wai Avenue, Beijing 100004, People's Republic of China
FEDERAL REPUBLIC OF GERMANY	Pergamon Press GmbH, Hammerweg 6, D-6242 Kronberg, Federal Republic of Germany
BRAZIL	Pergamon Editora Ltda, Rua Eça de Queiros, 346, CEP 04011, Paraiso, São Paulo, Brazil
AUSTRALIA	Pergamon Press Australia Pty Ltd., P.O. Box 544, Potts Point, NSW 2011, Australia
JAPAN	Pergamon Press, 8th Floor, Matsuoka Central Building, 1-7-1 Nishishinjuku, Shinjuku-ku, Tokyo 160, Japan
CANADA	Pergamon Press Canada Ltd., Suite 271, 253 College Street, Toronto, Ontario M5T 1R5, Canada

Library of Congress Cataloging in Publication Data

Poling, Alan D.
    Drug therapy for behavior disorders : an introduction / by Alan Poling, Kenneth D. Gadow, and James Cleary.
      p. cm. -- (Psychology practitioner guidebooks)
    Includes index.
    ISBN 0-08-034950-1:   --ISBN 0-08-034949-8 (pbk.):
    1. Psychotropic drugs. 2. Neuropsychopharmacology. I. Gadow, Kenneth D. II. Cleary, James Philip. III. Title. IV. Series.
    [DNLM: 1. Behavior—drug effects. 2. Mental Disorders—drug therapy. 3. Psychotropic Drugs—pharmacology. QV 77 768d]
RM315.P614 1990
615'.78—dc20
DNLM/DLC
for Library of Congress
                                    90-7233
                                       CIP

Printing: 1 2 3 4 5 6 7 8 9   Year: 1 2 3 4 5 6 7 8 9

Printed in the United States of America

The paper used in this publication meets the minimum requirements of American National Standard for Information Sciences—Permanence of Paper for Printed Library Materials, ANSI Z39.48-1984

Contents

Preface

Drug Therapy for Behavior Disorders: An Introduction was written to provide a nontechnical summary of the usual applications and effects of commonly prescribed psychotropic medications. Its intended audience is caregivers outside the medical professions. Of course, these caregivers are not directly responsible for decisions concerning psychotropic medications. Legal statutes dictate that such decisions are ultimately made by people specially trained in medicine and licensed to prescribe drugs, which include psychiatrists, pediatricians, and general practitioners. But it is grossly unfair to expect physicians to operate in isolation. Regardless of expertise, the person who writes prescriptions can provide optimal drug therapy for behavior disorders only if relevant feedback concerning a patient's response to medication is given. Caregivers outside the medical professions are often in an excellent position to provide such information, and its quality is apt to vary directly with their knowledge concerning the applications and effects of the drug in question. One reason for learning about drug therapy in behavior disorders is to be able to serve as a competent member of a drug assessment team. There are two other important reasons.

1. Psychotropic drugs are commonly used with many special populations and often produce significant and complex effects. Knowing the behavioral and physiological effects of these drugs helps in understanding clients and in meeting their unique needs. For instance, roughly 40% of patients treated with the antiepileptic drug phenytoin (Dilantin) develop excessive growth of the gums (gingival hyperplasia). Food particles often lodge in the gums, leading to inflammation. Because meticulous oral hygiene can reduce the severity of this problem, care providers should be aware of the problem and prepared to provide necessary assistance.

2. Drug therapy can alter the efficacy of nonpharmacological interventions by rendering the patient either more or less sensitive to collateral treatments. For instance, the behavior of a hospitalized manic patient may be largely insensitive to token reinforcement when he or she is not receiving lithium but very responsive when lithium is administered. There is growing awareness that optimal patient care characteristically involves a combination of pharmacological and behavioral treatments (e.g., Hersen, 1986).

One way to learn about pharmacological treatments is to consult the research literature. Unfortunately, the implications of published studies for clinical practice are sometimes difficult to discern, for three reasons. First, although the quality of published research has generally improved over time, many researchers continue to employ questionable methodologies, a practice which calls into question the soundness of their results and conclusions. Second, similar studies sometimes yield dissimilar findings or researchers' interpretations of particular findings differ, thus making it difficult for the reader to reach any strong conclusion. Third, the generality of reported findings is often difficult to determine. Drug A may be generally effective in treating behavior disorder B in population C, but what about other disorders and populations?

Despite the foregoing problems, it is possible to provide data-based summaries of the probable effects of various drug classes. *Drug Therapy for Behavior Disorders: An Introduction* does so in eight chapters. Chapter 1 provides an introduction. Chapter 2 offers a brief discussion of some fundamental concepts in pharmacology, a basic understanding of which aids in understanding chapters 4 to 8. Chapter 3 deals with measuring efficacy and untoward effects of medication. The emphasis here is practical: What strategies can caregivers use to aid physicians in evaluating medication? Chapters 4 through 7 summarize the effects of commonly encountered psychotropic medications: A separate chapter is devoted to each of four major drug classes (neuroleptics, sedative hypnotics and anxiolytics, stimulants, and antidepressant drugs and lithium). Following a common format, each chapter contains information on clinical applications, pharmacology, efficacy, untoward effects, and interactions with other drugs. Chapter 8 contains similar information about antiepileptic drugs. Although not typically used to manage behavior, these drugs are behaviorally active and are commonly encountered in special populations.

This book is intended to provide a simple and straightforward summary of how psychotropic medications are used and their probable effects. Emphasis is placed on common and characteristic applications; rare and experimental applications are ignored not because they are unimportant but because they are many and difficult to summarize. Drug-induced changes in behavior and in physiological status that are likely to be evident to caregivers are given first priority. Central nervous system (CNS) actions are mentioned where appropriate but are not considered at length. Because it is a small and practically oriented volume written for the nonspecialist, *Drug Therapy for Behavior Disorders: An Introduction* offers little for expert psychopharmacologists, who will recognize that we have painted with a broad brush, omitting much detail and ignoring many issues. But they will also be aware of more advanced sources of information and will have the training to make use of them. For the convenience of those of our readers who desire further information, a list of suggested readings for each chapter is provided at the end of the book. Some are a bit technical, but all are informative.

Chapter 1

Introduction

Human behavior is remarkably diverse; no two of us behave in precisely the same way. A wide range of behavior is tolerated in most societies, but certain actions cause trouble and force intervention. Consider the case of Harry. This hypothetical case is based on events that occur in schizophrenic disorders, although such disorders do not characteristically involve violence. Harry was born near Detroit and had a normal childhood. A good student and a fair athlete, he was popular through high school. Harry experienced most of the difficulties characteristic of youth, but his parents, teachers, and friends considered him generally warm and well adjusted. In the fall of 1987, Harry at 19 years of age enrolled in the sociology program at a local college. Shortly thereafter, his behavior began to change. At first, the change was subtle: Harry started spending more time alone in his dorm room, reading and listening to music. Over time, his attendance at classes and social events became increasingly sporadic and, on those rare occasions when he did venture out, he appeared preoccupied with the threat of a nuclear war initiated by Panama.

By the end of fall semester, Harry spent almost all of his time in his room and rarely spoke with other people. At home for the Christmas holiday, Harry avoided his family and old friends. When interactions did occur, they were often painful. This was the case on Christmas Eve, the traditional time for his family to decorate the tree. Instead of helping his parents and four siblings with the task, as he had always done, Harry chastised his family for constructing a graven image, then delivered a largely senseless monologue on the failings of humanity, his family in particular, and then on the Armageddon soon to come. Attempts to calm him failed. Harry eventually burst into tears, ran upstairs, and locked himself into a bedroom. He was quiet but caused no real problems on Christmas, and the family had a good holiday. Harry received his grades 2 days later. The arrival of three Fs, a D, and a B precipitated a long and bitter argument. When Harry's parents asked for an explanation of his poor performance, their son cursed them, something he had never done, and proclaimed them damned in a nuclear holocaust. He did so, however, in peculiar phrases: "You'll fry with me, won't you? Panama Canal, goodbye now. It wasn't like this before. They tell me, make us all deliver. Alpha, beta, gamma ray—fry your ass, blow your soul away. I'm out of here."

On New Year's Eve, Harry struck his youngest brother in the face with a wine bottle, cutting him badly. Understandably frightened and confused, Harry's parents called the police. Harry was taken to jail and then to the local hospital, where psychiatrists determined him to be in the active phase of a schizophrenic disorder, paranoid type.

Two years after Christmas 1987, Harry is living at home. He takes 15 mg of haloperidol (Haldol) every day. He makes no mention of nuclear war or Panama and has little trouble with his parents. He seldom interacts with other people, however, and most of his time is spent alone. Harry occasionally talks about getting a job or returning to school, but he has made little real progress toward either.

Why is Harry's case noteworthy? It is tempting to answer "because of his schizophrenia." While that is true, it is important to recognize that schizophrenia is a label for a set of troublesome behaviors that meet certain diagnostic criteria. Harry was labelled as schizophrenic because of what he did: Over time, his speech became progressively more bizarre, he failed to meet responsibilities, and his interactions with other people diminished. Finally, he violently assaulted a close relative. In essence, Harry caused a problem for himself and for those around him because he stopped behaving in desirable ways and began behaving in unacceptable ways. It was on the basis of his behavior and nothing more that he was diagnosed as schizophrenic. In a very real sense, schizophrenia is a behavior disorder.

As used in this book, *behavior disorders* include all conditions in which individuals cause a problem for themselves or for other people because they exhibit unacceptable behavior or fail to function appropriately. The disorder might be limited to one or two discrete responses, as in nighttime bedwetting (enuresis) or self-injurious face-slapping, or might involve a broad range of signs and symptoms, as in schizophrenia. The term behavior disorder emphasizes that what a person does or, more rarely, fails to do, constitutes a problem and provides the rationale for treatment. It implies nothing about the cause of the problem or the appropriateness of a given intervention. Historically, many psychologists have contended that the majority of behavior disorders are caused and maintained by environmental events and can be best treated by manipulating such variables. Many physicians, in contrast, have operated from the premise that most behavior disorders result from and can best be controlled by altering biomedical and physiological events. Neither position can be defended in the extreme (cf. Hersen, 1986).

Behavior disorders include conditions in which the primary manifestation is an undesirable subjective state (mood), because such states are characterized by specific overt behaviors. How, for example, can you determine whether a friend is depressed? Only by observing how he or she acts and talks about him- or herself. Unless there are extenuating circumstances, we are apt to label as depressed a person who suddenly stops going out, spends much time sleeping, and makes pessimistic and deprecating self-statements.

Psychiatrists and psychologists differentiate various kinds of behavior disorders, which they typically label collectively as "mental illnesses" or "psychiatric disorders." It is traditional in pharmacology and psychiatry to refer to all drugs that affect mood, thought processes, or overt behavior as *psychoactive*, and to those whose primary (or most clinically salient) feature is the production of such effects as *psychotropic*. The terms psychoactive drug and behaviorally active drug are rough synonyms, as are behavior-change medication and psychotropic medication.

BEHAVIOR-CHANGE
MEDICATION THROUGH
HISTORY

People severely handicapped by virtue of behavior disorders (including those who would currently be classified as schizophrenic) were recognized at least as early as 1400 B.C. (Julien, 1988). Through the centuries they have been pitied and cared for, scourged, prayed over, and used as a source of royal entertainment. Use of drug treatment for behavior disorders has a long history, but effective behavior-change medication first appeared in the present century. Prior to that time, the drugs used typically had laxative, diaphoretic, emetic, or sedative actions, which rendered patients less active and easier to manage. However, as discussed in chapter 3, nonselective suppression of behavior is not appropriate pharmacotherapy.

The modern era of psychopharmacology had its beginning in the 1950s with the widespread acceptance of chlorpromazine (Thorazine) in psychiatric practice, but some important advances were made earlier in the present century. For example, from 1910 to 1940 several studies of antiepileptic drugs (e.g., phenobarbital, phenytoin) and stimulants (e.g., benezedrine) appeared, and in 1949 the successful use of lithium in manic and agitated psychiatric patients was reported. In 1950, chlorpromazine was synthesized in France; its beneficial effects in psychiatric patients were first described in print in 1952. Chlorpromazine revolutionized psychiatry because it reduced the undesirable behaviors of most psychotic patients. Many studies have shown that chlorpromazine is generally effective for managing schizophrenia and other psychoses. However, not all psychotic individuals benefit from the drug; some improve without it, and all who receive it are at risk for developing motor dysfunctions and other deleterious side effects.

After the introduction of chlorpromazine, scores of other antipsychotic drugs were introduced into the market. In many cases, drug treatment sufficiently improved psychotic patients to allow them to leave hospitals. In fact in the first half of the twentieth century the number of patients in United States mental hospitals increased from approximately 150,000 to 500,000. In 1956, the first year that chlorpromazine was used widely in this country, this trend reversed itself and by 1970 the number of hospitalized patients had fallen to less than 350,000 (see Figure 1.1). The downward trend has continued to the present, although the rate of decline has slowed.

Interestingly, this reduction in the number of hospitalized patients has not resulted from a decrease in new admissions. Instead, effective behavior-change medication allows patients to leave the hospital after much briefer stays (Berger, 1978). Prior to the 1950s, patients with se-

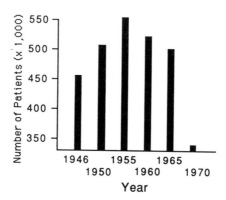

FIGURE 1.1. The number of resident patients in state and local mental hospitals in the United States in 1946, 1950, 1955, 1960, 1965, and 1970 as reported by Longo (1972). Chlorpromazine (Thorazine) and other effective behavior-change medications were introduced in the mid-1950s. At that time the number of resident patients, which had been steadily rising since the turn of the century, began to fall.

vere behavior disorders were commonly institutionalized for much of their lives.

The general effectiveness of neuroleptics firmly established psychotropic medication as a major weapon in the psychiatrists' armamentarium. But the search for better medications did not end, and many different psychotropic agents have been introduced in the ensuing years. Teasing apart the actions of various drugs demands research; from 1955 to the present time, tens of thousands of studies of behavior-change medication have appeared, forming the basis for the present-day science of psychopharmacology.

BEHAVIORAL AND PSYCHIATRIC DIAGNOSIS

On a descriptive level, behavior that creates a problem for patients can in most cases be divided into three general categories:

1. Behavior that is troublesome because of its topography (form). A child eating glass is an example; such behavior is a problem whenever and wherever it occurs.

2. Behavior that is troublesome because of its rate or intensity. A second-grader crying and asking to be hugged is an example. This is no problem if it occurs occasionally, but most parents would be understandably vexed if the request were repeated every 5 minutes. Behavior that fails to occur or occurs rarely can also be a problem, as when a child consistently fails to comply with a parent's commands.

3. Behavior that is troublesome because it occurs in inappropriate circumstances. Masturbating is an example; it is permissible in private but undesirable in public.

When much if not most of an individual's behavior is troublesome, it is common to consider the specific behavior problems as symptoms of a clinical disorder. Psychiatric diagnosis involves categorizing people according to the troublesome things they say and do. It is on this basis that the various forms of "mental illness" are distinguished. Although the distinction is no longer favored by some clinicians, the various forms of mental illness have for decades been divided on the basis of severity into psychoses and neuroses. *Psychoses* involve severe and pervasive behavioral problems. They are marked by pronounced functional impairment and often involve thought disorders (speaking and thinking illogically), hallucinations (reporting objects and events not actually present), and delusions (making statements obviously contrary to facts). Unusual affect (emotion) is also common. These symptoms are of course inferred on the basis of actual behavior.

Neuroses are less pervasive and debilitating than psychoses, although they can cause great suffering. Neuroses do not involve substantial loss of behavioral control by environmental events (i.e., "contact with reality" is maintained), and they often appear to be exaggerations of normal reactions. Like psychoses, neuroses are mental illnesses only in the sense that a part of their symptomatology involves reporting a world within the skin that differs from that familiar to most people. The "mind" has no physical status, it does not control behavior, and it cannot become ill. The CNS is real and does control behavior, and meaningful biological hypotheses of behavior disorders have been advanced. Despite this, at the present time it is not possible to explain most behavior disorders in terms of pathophysiological processes.

Mental disorder is an approximate synonym of mental illness. The American Psychiatric Association (APA) favors the former term and employs it in the *Diagnostic and Statistical Manual of Mental Disorders,* third edition, revised (DSM-III-R). DSM-III-R provides a widely used nosological system (nosology is the branch of medicine that deals with the classification of diseases). Box 1.1 considers the meaning of mental disorder as used in that volume (APA, 1987).

The complex diagnostic system presented in DSM-III-R requires that each patient be assessed on a number of dimensions or "axes." These are (a) clinical syndromes, (b) developmental disorders and personality disorders, (c) physical disorders and conditions, (d) severity of psychosocial stressors, and (e) global assessment of functioning. The first three axes determine the official DSM-III-R diagnosis and the last two provide supplemental information. Table 1.1 lists major Axis I and II categories, each of which includes a number of subcategories not listed.

To provide some notion of how DSM-III-R categories are applied, we consider the diagnostic criteria for schizophrenia. (Only the general category of schizophrenia is considered, although DSM-III-R deals with a number of subcategories.) The manual lists six diagnostic criteria for schizophrenia, and each must be present for the diagnosis to be assigned. These criteria are listed in Table 1.2. Although these criteria are further described in DSM-III-R, even with book in hand they are rather vague. As Lickey and Gordon (1983) emphasize, "A reliable system of diagnosis will achieve at least two goals. First, it will clearly define each illness by specifying its symptoms. Second, it will specify the methods for determining whether a patient has a particular symptom" (p. 39).

DSM-III-R falls somewhat short on both counts. Nonetheless, this nosological system is adequate to allow for meaningful communication among researchers and clinicians, and to aid in clinical practice. For example, psychiatric diagnosis is related to the likelihood that a patient

Box 1.1. What are mental disorders?

In DSM-III-R each of the mental disorders is conceptualized as a clinically significant behavioral or psychological syndrome or pattern that occurs in a person and that is associated with present distress (a painful symptom) or disability (impairment in one or more important areas of functioning) or with a significantly increased risk of suffering death, pain, disability, or an important loss of freedom. In addition, this syndrome or pattern must not be merely an expectable response to a particular event, for example, the death of a loved one. Whatever its original cause, it must currently be considered a manifestation of a behavioral, psychological, or biological dysfunction in the person. Neither deviant behavior, whether political, religious, or sexual, nor conflicts that are primarily between the individual and society are mental disorders unless the deviance or conflict is a symptom of a dysfunction in the person, as described.

There is no assumption that each mental disorder is a discrete entity with sharp boundaries (discontinuity) between it and other mental disorders or between it and no mental disorder. For example, there has been a continuing controversy concerning whether severe depressive disorder and mild depressive disorder differ from each other qualitatively (discontinuity between diagnostic entities) or quantitatively (a difference on a severity continuum).

A common misconception is that a classification of mental disorders classifies people, when actually what are being classified are disorders that people have. . . . Another misconception is that all people described as having the same mental disorder are alike in all important ways. Although all the people described as having the same mental disorder have at least the defining features of the disorder, they may well differ in other important respects that may affect clinical management and outcome.

Note: From American Psychiatric Association: *Diagnostic and Statistical Manual of Mental Disorders, Third Edition, Revised,* pp. xxii–xxiii, Washington, DC, American Psychiatric Association, 1987. Reprinted by permission.

will benefit from treatment with a particular type of medication. A diagnosis of schizophrenia, for instance, suggests that an antipsychotic drug such as thioridazine (Mellaril) might be useful, whereas an antidepressant or a stimulant would not be helpful.

There is, however, considerable latitude in the range of conditions that respond to a given drug. As Baldessarini (1985b) notes:

Antipsychotic drugs exert beneficial effects in virtually all classes of psychotic illness, and, contrary to a common misconception, are not selective for schizophrenia. Moreover, antidepressant drugs that are especially beneficial in severe depression can also exert useful effects on less

Table 1.1. DSM-III-R Major Categories

Axis I: Clinical Syndromes
Disorders usually first evident in infancy, childhood, or adolescence:
  Developmental disorders
  Disruptive behavior disorders
  Anxiety disorders of childhood or adolescence
  Eating disorders
  Gender identity disorders
  Tic disorders
  Elimination disorders
  Speech disorders not elsewhere classified
  Other disorders of infancy, childhood, or adolescence
Organic mental disorders:
  Dementias arising in the senium and presenium
  Psychoactive substance-induced organic mental disorders
  Organic mental disorders associated with physical disorders or conditions, or whose
    etiology is unknown
Psychoactive substance use disorders
Schizophrenia
Delusional (paranoid) disorders
Psychotic disorders not elsewhere classified
Mood disorders:
  Bipolar disorders
  Depressive disorders
Anxiety disorders
Somatoform disorders
Dissociative disorders
Sexual disorders:
  Paraphilias
  Sexual dysfunctions
  Other sexual disorders
Sleep disorders:
  Dyssomnias
  Parasomnias
Factitious disorders
Impulse control disorders not elsewhere classified
Adjustment disorders

Axis II: Developmental and Personality Disorders
Developmental disorders:
  Mental retardation
  Pervasive developmental disorders
  Specific developmental disorders
Personality disorders:
  Cluster A (paranoid, schizoid, schizotypal)
  Cluster B (antisocial, borderline, histrionic, narcissistic)

Note: From American Psychiatric Association: *Diagnostic and Statistical Manual of Mental Disorders, Third Edition, Revised*, pp. 3–9. Washington, DC, American Psychiatric Association, 1987.

severe depressive syndromes and on conditions that are not obviously depressive in nature (e.g., panic attacks, eating disorders, chronic pain, obsessive compulsive disorders). Thus, in general, psychotropic drugs are not disease specific; they provide clinical benefit from specific syndromes or complexes of symptoms (p. 389).

Table 1.2. Diagnostic Criteria for Schizophrenia

A. Presence of characteristic psychotic symptoms as indicated by 1, 2, or 3 below:
   1. two of the following:
      a. delusions
      b. prominent hallucinations
      c. incoherence or marked loosening of associations
      d. catatonic behavior
      e. flat or grossly inappropriate affect
   2. bizarre delusions
   3. prominent hallucinations of a voice with content having no apparent relation to depression or elation or commenting on the person's behavior, or two or more voices conversing with each other
B. Deteriorations from previous level of functioning in such areas as work, social relations, and self-care.
C. Other conditions (schizoaffective disorder and mood disorder with psychotic features) have been ruled out.
D. Duration of at least 6 months. Prodromal and residual phases are also described.
E. Not due to an organic mental disorder.
F. If a history of autistic disorder is present, schizophrenia is diagnosed only if prominent delusions or hallucinations occur.

Note: From American Psychiatric Association: *Diagnostic and Statistical Manual of Mental Disorders, Third Edition, Revised,* pp. 194–195, Washington, DC, American Psychiatric Association, 1987. Reprinted by permission.

Chapters 3 through 7 in this book consider the syndromes and symptoms that typically respond favorably to treatment with various classes of psychotropic medications.

CONCLUDING COMMENT

Behavior disorders take many forms and range in seriousness from mildly disconcerting to life threatening. Psychotropic medications are effective in treating many behavior disorders, and the availability of these medications has revolutionized psychiatry. There is no doubt that millions of patients have derived significant benefit from psychotropic medications. Nonetheless, psychotropic drugs are not panaceas. Some patients with behavior disorders do not respond favorably to any psychotropic medication, and all patients who receive psychotropic medications are at risk for experiencing adverse reactions. Given this, pharmacological interventions should be tailored to individual patients, and their effects monitored carefully.

Chapter 2
Principles of Pharmacology

A drug is any chemical that affects living processes. Although some drugs come from plants and animals, most are derived from synthetic substances. The nomenclature used to describe drugs is rather confusing. All drugs have a chemical name, which provides a description of the molecule according to rules outlined in *Chemical Abstracts*. In addition to its chemical name, a new drug is usually given a code name by its manufacturer. If the drug is developed for clinical use, the drug will be given a United States Adopted Name (USAN) by a panel of experts. The USAN is a nonproprietary name and is often referred to as the generic name of the drug. Some pharmacologists contend, however, that this usage is incorrect and that generic names properly refer to chemical or pharmacological classes of drugs, not to individual medications (e.g., Blaschke, Nies & Mamelok, 1985). When a drug is admitted to the *United States Pharmacopeia*, which lists therapeutic agents approved for use in the United States, the USAN becomes the official name. Nonproprietary (or generic) names are commonly used in the clinical literature and for this reason are used in this text.

After a drug is given an official name, it is also assigned a proprietary name (or trade name) by the manufacturer. These names are protected by trademark laws, are usually easy to pronounce, and may suggest a drug's therapeutic application. Trade names are typically capitalized when they appear in print. In this book, the trade name appears in parentheses following the first citation of the generic name. A drug manufacturer patents a newly formulated agent and controls the right to manufacture it for 17 years. When the period of patent protection expires, any drug company can manufacture the drug and sell it either by its nonproprietary (generic) name or by a different trade name. Medications marketed by several manufacturers may have several trade names.

Drugs are classified in many ways, none of which is entirely satisfactory. The most common classification scheme, and that adopted in this book, is according to therapeutic usage. For example, antidepressants reduce or eliminate the subjective feelings and troublesome behaviors that lead to a clinical diagnosis of depression. Although the members of a given therapeutic class may differ in significant ways, they all share common properties, and it is convention in pharmacology to emphasize a small number of prototypes in describing the effects of particular drug classes. An extensive listing of selected psychotropic and antiepileptic drugs by generic (nonproprietary) name, with corresponding trade name and drug classification, appears in Appendix A.

PHARMACOKINETICS

Pharmacokinetics refers to the absorption, distribution, biotransformation, and excretion of drug molecules. These processes determine, in large part, the intensity and duration of drug effects. *Absorption* is the process whereby drug molecules enter the bloodstream. *Distribution* involves the movement of drug molecules through the bloodstream to the site of action, the place where drug molecules affect protoplasm to produce an effect. *Biotransformation* refers to the changes in the structure of drug molecules characteristically produced by enzymatic action in the liver. Most drugs are converted into inactive metabolites, but some are changed to an active form. *Excretion* is the process responsible for the removal of drug molecules and metabolites from the body, usually in the urine.

Absorption

A drug must enter the body before it can be absorbed, and the manner in which it does so is termed the *route of administration*. Although intravenous and intramuscular routes are occasionally used for special purposes, psychotropic drugs are usually taken orally. This is a convenient and economical route of administration and is usually safer than other routes. To be absorbed after ingestion, drugs in tablet or capsule form must dissolve in the fluids of the stomach or the intestine. They then pass through the cells that line the wall of the digestive tract and into the capillaries of the veins that lead from the stomach and small intestine to the liver.

Drugs differ dramatically with respect to how readily they are absorbed following ingestion. As a rule, molecules that are very *lipid-soluble* (i.e., readily combine with fats, which are present in cellular membranes) cross membranes, and hence pass into and out of the bloodstream, more readily than drugs that are less lipid-soluble. Molecules that are not electrically charged (i.e., those that are un-ionized) also cross membranes more readily than electrically charged (ionized) molecules. With many drugs, the proportion of molecules that are ionized depends on the relative acidity/alkalinity (pH) of the medium in which they are found (e.g., gastric fluid). Hence, changing gastric pH can affect absorption. A few drugs (e.g., insulin) are inactivated by stomach enzymes, and others do not pass readily through cell membranes and consequently do not gain entry into the bloodstream. Even for a drug that is absorbed relatively well, the amount that will enter the blood stream may be difficult to estimate accurately. Individuals differ with respect to their natural speed of absorption, which (as discussed above) is also influenced by stomach and intestinal pH (acidity/alkalinity) and the presence of food or other drugs in the gut. Because food alters absorption, many medications are taken between meals. The usual exceptions are those agents that cause gastric upset if taken on an empty stomach.

The rate of absorption is determined, in part, by the form in which the drug is administered. Liquids are usually absorbed more readily than solids, although the two dosage forms sometimes are used interchangeably. Particulars of manufacture, such as the thickness of the pill coating, type of filler substances, and hardness of the tablet also alter the rate of absorption. Therefore, different brands of the same drug may be absorbed at different rates. This can be of clinical significance because the amount of drug in the blood is related to therapeutic response.

In some cases, manufacturers intentionally prepare drugs in a form that slows absorption. For example, CIBA Pharmaceuticals markets methylphenidate (Ritalin) in the form of regular and sustained-release (Ritalin SR) tablets. Active drug is more slowly absorbed from the sustained-release tablets, which prolongs the duration of drug effects (Birhamer, Greenhill, Cooper, Fried, & Maminski, 1989). Because chewing sustained-release Ritalin tablets speeds absorption, patients are advised to swallow them whole.

Distribution

Once in the bloodstream, drug molecules are distributed throughout the body, but they characteristically produce their effects at localized *sites of action*. Psychotropic drugs, for example, alter the functioning of cells located in the CNS. To reach these sites of action, molecules pass from the small arteries to the capillaries, then through the capillary walls to the extracellular fluid, where they diffuse and eventually contact the neurons in the brain. At a given time, only a tiny fraction of the total amount of drug molecules in the body is at the site of action.

The molecules of many drugs combine with large protein molecules in the blood in a process called *protein binding*. Protein-bound molecules are unable to pass out of the bloodstream and do not reach the site of action, but this process is not irreversible. As unbound molecules pass out of the bloodstream, bound molecules are released so that the ratio of bound to unbound molecules in the blood remains roughly constant. Although the maximal effect of a drug is reduced by protein binding, the process prolongs the effect of the drug by creating a reservoir of bound drug molecules that are released over time (Briant, 1978). The concentration of drug molecules in fat or muscle cells (which occurs with some medications) has the same effect.

The passage of certain drugs out of the bloodstream and into the brain is impeded by glial cells that closely surround the capillaries of the brain. The term *blood–brain barrier* is used to emphasize the difficulty with which drugs enter the brain, but the term has no precise structural referent. Because most psychotropic drugs are lipid-soluble, they cross membranes readily and enter the brain with relative ease.

Biotransformation

As they pass through the body, most drugs are changed into new compounds termed *metabolites*. Substances within the cells of the liver, called *enzymes*, initiate and facilitate the chemical reactions that transform drugs into metabolites. In most cases an active drug is metabolized into a substance (or substances) that is water soluble and can be excreted through the kidneys. Some drugs, however, are not metabolized and pass from the body unchanged. Others are transformed into active metabolites.

Excretion

Drugs and their metabolites are removed from the body primarily by the actions of the kidneys. Although most drugs exit from the body as water-soluble molecules dissolved in urine, significant quantities of certain drugs are excreted in feces or in exhaled air. Measurable amounts may also be present in sweat, saliva, tears, or the milk of nursing mothers. The rate of excretion of some drugs is affected by the pH of the urine. Drugs that are bases are generally excreted more rapidly when the urine is acidic, whereas acidic drugs are more rapidly excreted in basic urine. Many other variables influence the rate of inacti-vation and elimination of drugs. Among them are genotype, age, drug history, and liver or kidney disease.

Time-Course of Action

With psychotropic medications, a relationship clearly exists between the effects of the drug and its concentration in the body (e.g., in blood). When a drug is given on a single occasion (i.e., acutely), the level of drug in the blood and the effects it produces will vary as a function of time since administration. Each substance has a characteristic *time-course of action*, which refers to the magnitude and direction of its physiolog-ical and behavioral actions as a function of time since administration. The time-course of action for a given drug is determined by its physical properties, the dose administered, the route of administration, and or-ganismic variables (e.g., age, health, genotype, drug history) that alter the body's response to the drug.

Just as the rate of disappearance of a radioactive isotope is expressed as the time needed for 50% of it to decay (the half-life), the rate of disappearance of drug molecules is described in terms of its biological half-life. The *half-life* of a drug is determined by measuring the amount of time required for a given blood level to decline by 50%. With many drugs, this value does not change significantly as a function of initial drug blood level or dosage, and such drugs are described as having *linear* (or first-order) *kinetics*. For such drugs, a constant fraction of drug is eliminated per unit time. Table 2.1 shows how a hypothetical drug with a half-life of 2 hours would be eliminated across time. In this table, it is assumed that the drug was administered intravenously, which would result in peak blood levels being reached immediately.

Some drugs have *nonlinear* kinetics, which means that the mecha-nisms that eliminate them can become saturated, causing the relative rate of elimination to decrease (and the apparent half-life to increase) with dosage and concentration. In such cases, there is a range of ap-parent half-lives for any individual, each affected by the dose and the initial concentration at which it is measured.

Table 2.1. Percent of Maximum Drug Blood Level Following Intravenous Administration of a Hypothetical Drug with Linear Kinetics and a Half-Life of 2 Hours

	Hours Since Injection					
	0	2	4	6	8	10
Drug blood level (%)	100	50	25	12.5	6.25	3.13

Even for drugs with linear kinetics, the rate of elimination varies across individuals as a function of genetics, physiological characteristics, and exposure to that drug and others (i.e., drug history). Therefore, half-life values are expressed only within rather broad ranges. Those values are, however, of therapeutic importance. For example, a medication should be administered approximately once per half-life to maintain stable blood levels. Because it takes approximately five half-lives after the first administration to reach a stable blood level, evaluations of drug efficacy prior to that time will be inconclusive.

If a drug is taken in more rapidly than it can be inactivated, blood levels and overt effects increase over time. This phenomenon, known as *accumulation*, can be a clinically significant problem, especially with long-acting drugs with variable half-lives.

DOSE-DEPENDENT DRUG EFFECTS

The effects of all drugs are dose-dependent: the amount of drug that is administered determines both qualitative and quantitative aspects of its effects. At very low doses, all drugs fail to produce observable effects; and at high enough doses, all drugs produce toxic (harmful) reactions. Symptomatic changes observed between these end points typically are of greatest therapeutic interest, although toxic effects resulting from an excessively high dosage are always important.

Recommended dosage limits, both minimum and maximum, are available for all psychotropic drugs. In clinical practice, the physician typically starts with a relatively small amount of medication, which is gradually increased until the desired response is achieved, the maximum suggested dosage is reached, or significant untoward reactions appear. This procedure is sometimes referred to as *titration*. Chapter 3 describes strategies for monitoring therapeutic and undesired effects of psychotropic drugs.

Medication is typically measured in milligrams (mg). One mg is approximately 1/28,000 of an ounce. Because people vary considerably in body size, it is convention among clinical researchers to describe and prescribe doses in terms of units of drug (mg) per unit of body weight (kg). A kg equals about 2.2 pounds. Thus, if a 176-pound (80-kg) person received 50 mg of drug A each day, the daily dose would be 6.25 mg/kg (50/80). Although the mg/kg designation is more precise, recommended doses are often expressed in terms of absolute amount of medication administered per day (mg/day), with adult and child doses listed separately.

With some drugs, the amount of medication administered has little relationship to the level of drug in the blood. For those agents, a more useful measure than mg/kg/day (or mg/day) is one that indicates how much drug is in the blood, which is often expressed as micrograms (mcg or μg) of drug per milliliter (mL) of blood. With the exception of lithium (see chapter 7), it is uncommon to measure blood levels of psychotropic agents. But, as described in chapter 8, blood level determinations play an important role in therapy with antiepileptic medications.

Within reason, the amount of medication required to produce a therapeutic response is unimportant. For example, the usual antipsychotic dose range for haloperidol is 6 to 20 mg/day, whereas the recommended dose of chlorpromazine is 300 to 800 mg/day (Baldessarini, 1985b). Haloperidol is more potent (when used precisely, *potency* refers to the amount of drug required to produce a given effect), but not necessarily better. Potent drugs may appear especially powerful and therefore useful, but the value of any medication depends on how much it benefits a patient at the most effective dose (i.e., its *efficacy*), not on the absolute or relative size of that dose.

TOLERANCE AND DEPENDENCE

Tolerance, shown graphically in Figure 2.1, occurs when repeated (i.e., chronic) administration of a given dose produces a smaller effect or when a higher dose is required to produce the same effect. All drugs have multiple effects, and tolerance does not develop to each of them at the same rate or to the same degree. For example, tolerance usually develops to the drowsiness associated with neuroleptic medications, but rarely develops to their antipsychotic actions.

In some cases, repeated exposure to one drug decreases a person's reactivity to another drug. This phenomenon, termed cross-tolerance, generally occurs for drugs that have similar pharmacological properties.

The mechanisms responsible for the development of tolerance are not completely known. When repeated administrations of a given drug increase the rate of elimination, this is called *metabolic* (or kinetic) tolerance. Metabolic tolerance usually is caused by an increased production of the enzymes within liver cells that are responsible for biotransformation, a process known as *microsomal enzyme induction.* *Pharmacodynamic* (or cellular) tolerance occurs when a given level of drug at the site of action produces weaker responses on subsequent exposures. In pharmacodynamic tolerance, the cells of the nervous system

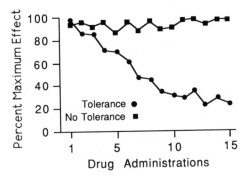

FIGURE 2.1. Hypothetical effects of repeated administrations of a drug that produced tolerance (circles) and another to which tolerance did not develop (squares). When tolerance occurs, the effects of a drug lessen with repeated administrations, although the rapidity and magnitude of this effect may vary.

somehow compensate for the presence of the medication. Metabolic and pharmacodynamic tolerance appear together with certain drugs.

Tolerance to therapeutic drug effects can be an important clinical management problem, because repeated dosage increases may lead to drug levels that cause serious adverse reactions. In the treatment of hyperactivity, for example, clinicians have described individual cases that showed a highly favorable response to one stimulant (e.g., methylphenidate) but later had to be switched to another (e.g., dextroamphetamine) because tolerance developed to the initial drug (Eichlseder, 1985). The general strategy of within-class drug substitutions as a solution to problems of tolerance to one agent is, however, effective only when cross-tolerance is not a problem.

Repeated exposure to some drugs produces physical dependence. A person is *physically dependent* on a drug if a withdrawal (or abstinence) syndrome appears when exposure to the drug is terminated. The withdrawal syndrome involves changes in physiological status (e.g., seizures), overt behavior (e.g., increased drug seeking), or subjective state (e.g., depression). The specific signs and symptoms that constitute the withdrawal syndrome vary in kind and intensity with drug type and dosage regimen.

One explanation of the withdrawal syndrome is that continuous exposure to the drug causes a physiological adaptation (e.g., changes in cell membranes), which results from the activation of systems that compensate for the presence of the drug in the body. These compensatory systems continue to operate for a time when the drug is withdrawn, and it is their action that leads to the withdrawal syndrome.

Consistent with this analysis (which also accounts for pharmacody-namic tolerance) is the observation that physiological responses during withdrawal are characteristically in the opposite direction from the re-sponses produced by the drug. For that reason, they are sometimes called *rebound effects*. Tolerance may, however, occur in the absence of marked physical dependence, and tolerance and physical dependence do not always develop in parallel (National Institute on Drug Abuse, 1978).

Psychological dependence is a term used in many ways, but it generally refers to a situation in which a person regularly self-administers a par-ticular drug. Psychological dependence in this sense is not necessarily harmful. For instance, many people regularly self-administer caffeine without hurting themselves or anyone else. When drug use becomes harmful and compulsive, it is often termed addiction. *Drug addiction* refers to a "behavioral pattern of drug use, characterized by over-whelming involvement with the use of the drug (compulsive use), the securing of its supply, and a high tendency to relapses after with-drawal" (Jaffee, 1985, p. 533). Physical dependence frequently accom-panies drug addiction, but this is not always the case: A person can be addicted to a drug without being physically dependent and vice versa.

MECHANISMS OF DRUG ACTION

Psychotropic drugs produce their therapeutic effects by affecting the functioning of nerve cells in the brain, which is a wondrously complex organ. The human brain contains approximately 20 billion neurons, each of which may share up to 100,000 *synapses* (connections) with other neurons (Zimbardo, 1988). Understanding how such a complex system works and how it is affected by drugs is a Herculean task. Nonethe-less, in recent years much has been learned. It is now known that the transmission of information in the CNS is an electrochemical process largely controlled by substances called *neurotransmitters*, which are pro-duced in neurons (nerve cells). Information is passed along individual nerve cells by the movement of charged particles across the cell mem-brane into and out of cells, which produces a wave of electrical activity (termed the *neuronal impulse)* that moves down the length of the neu-ron. This activity can lead to the release of a neurotransmitter, a chem-ical produced and stored in the neuron. Neurotransmitter molecules cross the fluid-filled gap (synaptic cleft) between neurons and interact with receptors on the membrane of the next neuron. Receptors are parts of a cell (e.g., proteins, nucleic acids, lipids of cell membranes) to which neurotransmitters bind chemically. Individual receptors are sensitive to specific neurotransmitters. Receptor–neurotransmitter interactions affect the probability that a neuronal impulse will be initiated. If the probability is increased, the effect is excitatory; if decreased, it is inhibitory. All neurons are affected by excitatory and inhibitory processes and the exquisite beauty of the nervous system is maintained by this delicate balance between excitation and inhibition (Julien, 1988).

Many substances are known to function as neurotransmitters, and the list grows each year. Among the best-studied neurotransmitters are norepinephrine, serotonin, dopamine, acetylcholine, and gamma aminobutyric acid (GABA). Drugs can affect neurotransmission in several ways, including the following:

1. By altering the synthesis (production in the body) of the neurotransmitter
2. By interfering with the storage of the neurotransmitter
3. By altering the release of the neurotransmitter
4. By interfering with the inactivation of the neurotransmitter (by enzymes or reuptake)
5. By interacting with receptors

The neuropharmacological actions of some psychotropic drugs are specifiable and relate to their clinical effectiveness. For instance, neuroleptics such as thioridazine (Mellaril) and chlorpromazine (Thorazine) appear to produce their antipsychotic effects by blocking receptors that respond to the neurotransmitter dopamine. A lock-and-key analogy is often used to explain this action: the receptor is envisioned as a lock, and molecules of dopamine and neuroleptics as similar but not identical keys. The dopamine key matches the receptor lock perfectly and will unlock it, thereby affecting the neuron on which the receptor is located. The neuroleptic key, in contrast, matches the receptor lock imperfectly: The neuroleptic key will enter the lock, but will not unlock it. Therefore, when neuroleptic molecules combine with dopamine receptors, cellular activity is not directly affected. But, just as ill-fitting keys prevent matching keys from entering and opening locks, neuroleptic molecules prevent dopamine molecules from combining with receptors and affecting the activity of the neuron. The end result is a reduction in neuronal activity in parts of the brain where dopamine is the neurotransmitter.

Blocking dopaminergic activity with neuroleptic medication provides relief of symptoms in most patients diagnosed as schizophrenic. Moreover, prolonged exposure to drugs that increase dopaminergic activity (e.g., amphetamine) produces changes in behavior that resemble those characteristic of schizophrenia. These findings led to the speculation that schizophrenia resulted from metabolic errors leading to either

(a) overproduction of dopamine in the limbic system or cortex of the brain or (b) production of an endogenous amphetamine-like compound (Baldessarini, 1985a). Such dopamine models of schizophrenia continue to be popular, but attempts to document metabolic differences in humans diagnosed as schizophrenic have yielded inconclusive results (Baldessarini, 1985b). Moreover, genetic studies have suggested that inheritance can account for only a portion of the causation of schizophrenia. In view of these considerations, biological models of schizophrenia based on inborn errors of metabolism that lead to overproduction of dopamine or an amphetamine-like substance are not fully adequate. Nor, for that matter, are other models of the disorder.

At present, it is not possible to explain behavior disorders fully in terms of biochemical mechanisms. We have at best a gross and incomplete understanding of how the brain functions and how it changes during behavior disorders, and of the mechanisms through which medications alter the process. In subsequent chapters, the neuropharmacological actions of various drug classes are briefly described, but these actions are in a practical sense far less important than the changes in mood, overt behavior, and thought processes produced by these agents. For that reason, it is these effects, not neuropharmacological actions, that are emphasized. Readers interested in the neuropharmacological actions of psychotropic drugs and biochemical models of mental illness are referred to reviews by Baldessarini (1985b), Clark and del Guidice (1978), Lipton, Di Mascio, and Killam (1978), and van Praag (1981).

DRUG INTERACTIONS

When a patient receives two or more psychoactive drugs, to treat either the same or different disorders, the practice is called *polypharmacy*. Polypharmacy is quite common. The term *multiple-drug therapy* is usually restricted to the prescribing of two or more drugs for the same condition. The latter practice is generally unwarranted unless (a) the medications have different mechanisms of action and (b) the clinical utility of the two in combination is clearly superior to that of either when used singly. Despite this restriction, multiple-drug therapy is surprisingly common.

At a descriptive level, the effects of two drugs given together can be additive, infraadditive, or supraadditive (synergistic). When the effects of two drugs are *additive,* their combined effects approximately equal a simple summation of their individual effects. For example, if at a given dose Drug A increased blood pressure by 10% and Drug B increased it by 20%, the two doses given in combination would increase blood pressure by 30% if their effects were additive. Infraadditive effects are less than additive (a blood pressure increase of less than 30% in our example), whereas supraadditive effects are greater than additive (over 30% increase in our example).

If the presence of one drug significantly alters the effects of another, a drug interaction has occurred. Drugs can interact through a sizeable number of mechanisms. In some cases, known collectively as pharmacokinetic interactions, one agent alters the absorption, distribution, biotransformation or excretion of another. Consider, for example, a situation in which Drug A inhibits the biotransformation of Drug B, which is inactivated by liver enzymes. This would result in higher blood levels of Drug B, which could produce an increased level of efficacy or toxicity or both. If, in contrast, Drug A induced (increased the level of) the enzymes that inactivate Drug B, the result would be a decrease in the blood levels and the effects of Drug B.

In addition to pharmacokinetic interactions, drugs can interact by directly affecting the same physiological system, either by acting in parallel or opposite directions, or by altering different physiological systems that have a common end point. Although the possibility of harmful drug interactions should never be ignored when polypharmacy is practiced, many drugs do not interact in a clinically significant way. Moreover, polypharmacy is often unavoidable when a patient has two or more disorders, each of which requires a different medication.

UNTOWARD EFFECTS

Although they would be of great value, there are no psychotropic drugs that selectively eliminate the target symptoms of behavior disorders without affecting the patient in other ways. All psychotropic drugs are potentially harmful. Ironically, adverse reactions may result from the same mechanism of action responsible for the therapeutic response. For example, blockade of dopamine receptors in certain parts of the brain appears to produce the clinical benefits associated with neuroleptics. This same action in other areas of the brain leads to serious disturbances of motor activity (see chapter 4). Because neuroleptics block dopamine receptors wherever they are located, the two effects cannot be independent. However, not all adverse reactions to neuroleptics involve dopamine. To varying degrees, individual neuroleptic drugs affect neurons where the neurotransmitter is acetylcholine, histamine, or norepinephrine. These actions, as well as the blockade of two subtypes (D_1 and D_2) of dopamine receptors, produce a wide array of behavioral and somatic effects. As discussed in the next chapter, deciding whether a given patient should receive a particular neuroleptic, or any other psychotropic medication, requires a careful cost–benefit analysis based on expected and observed therapeutic and adverse reactions.

Sources of Drug Information

Several good general sources of information about psychotropic and other psychoactive drugs include *The United States Pharmacopeia Dispensing Information* (two volumes), the *American Hospital Formulary Service*, *AMA Drug Evaluations*, *The Medical Letter*, *Clin-Alert*, *Rational Drug Therapy*, *The United States Pharmacopeia*, and *The National Formulary*. The *Physicians' Desk Reference* (PDR) is a commonly used source of drug information, but not the best one. The manufacturers whose drugs are described in the PDR support the volume, and the information contained is essentially identical to that which appears in the drug package inserts.

CONCLUDING COMMENT

The basic principles of pharmacology are well established and form a foundation for understanding the actions of psychotropic drugs. Those actions are, however, remarkably complex. At the present time, it is not possible to explain completely the beneficial effects of psychotropic medications in terms of their physiological actions. Moreover, it is not possible to predict accurately the specific behavioral effects of a given medication in a particular patient. Because of this, accurate assessment of patients' responses to medications is a critical element in the pharmacological management of behavior disorders.

Chapter 3

Measuring Efficacy and Untoward Effects

Behavior-change medications are prescribed to deal with problems. A patient receives such a drug because something she or he is (or, more rarely, is not) doing is deemed troublesome by the patient or by another legitimately interested person, perhaps a parent or spouse. Consider the case of John, a 9-year-old boy attending fourth grade. John's school grades are poor. His teacher reports that he is restless and impulsive, is always "on the go," gets along poorly with other children, and has a short attention span. At home, John frequently is aggressive toward his younger sister and is restive and inattentive. John's troublesome behaviors eventually cause his parents to seek professional help. After several visits to a local children's hospital, a pediatrician makes the diagnosis of Attention-deficit Hyperactivity Disorder (ADHD) and initiates treatment with methylphenidate (Ritalin) at a daily dosage of 30 mg (15 mg morning and noon).

As Sprague and Werry (1971) pointed out, every prescription of a psychotropic medication is in essence an experiment in which the physician hypothesizes that administering a specific drug will produce a desired change in one or more aspects of the patient's behavior. In the context of scientific research, a sound clinical drug study meets four minimal requirements: (a) medication must be administered according to the treatment plan, (b) drug effects must be adequately measured, (c) data analysis must be adequate to detect clinically important changes in behavior, and (d) conditions must be arranged so that observed changes in behavior can be attributed with confidence to the drug. These same requirements are important in the practical evaluation of medication, although assessment procedures employed outside research settings rarely meet the rigorous methodological standards advocated

23

by scientists. John's parents and physician are not interested in conducting a study worthy of presentation to the scientific community, but only in determining whether methylphenidate is an appropriate treatment for the boy. The purpose of the present chapter is to consider issues related to whether a particular patient is deriving benefit from medication, not to discuss research issues in clinical drug evaluation. The latter topic is extensively covered elsewhere (e.g., Gadow & Poling, 1986).

THERAPEUTIC AND SIDE EFFECTS

If John benefits from treatment with methylphenidate, those aspects of his behavior that constitute problems must improve when the drug is given. Moreover, the drug must not significantly impair other aspects of his functioning or his health. When a drug is used therapeutically, the desired action is termed the *therapeutic effect*. Any other action is a *side effect*. Side effects may be adverse, beneficial, or innocuous, but untoward responses typically are of greatest interest. Adverse drug reactions include (a) toxic effects due to overmedication, (b) common side effects that appear at therapeutic dosages and (c) idiosyncratic side effects (e.g., allergic reactions) that are not clearly related to dose. Side effects vary from mildly annoying to life-threatening. Their nature and severity depend on the drug in question and the dosage prescribed. Side effects of specific medications are described in chapters 4 through 8. In general, there are four strategies for dealing with side effects: (1) dosage reduction, (2) drug change, (3) adjunctive medication, and (4) drug discontinuation. In most cases, side effects can be reduced to tolerable levels without resorting to drug discontinuation.

OUTCOME MEASURES

Psychotropic medication is effective if it changes behavior in the desired way without inducing significant adverse reactions. Anyone concerned with evaluating the efficacy of a psychotropic medication will profit from asking three questions: (1) How will the patient's behavior change if treatment is effective? (2) How can improvement in the patient's behavior (i.e., therapeutic effects) best be detected? (3) How can potential side effects (behavioral impairment as well as somatic complaints) be detected? Unfortunately, in many cases these questions are easier to ask than to answer.

Let us return to John. How can one ascertain whether methylphenidate is producing the intended effect? To answer that question, one must first decide what the target symptoms are and then consider how they can be measured. With respect to John, the desired effect is management of ADHD. But what is that? Not a thing, but a diagnostic label assigned to patients who are inattentive, impulsive, and motorically active. These terms describe behaviors that share certain characteristics. For example, a child might be considered inattentive if she or he did not stay with one activity for very long, did not follow directions, and required repeated reminders to do things. Ultimately, it is these behaviors (symptoms) that are targeted for change. To determine whether John benefits from treatment, one must directly or indirectly measure these target behaviors both on and off medication.

Many different procedures can be used to quantify target behaviors. Regardless of the strategy adopted, the reliability, validity, and sensitivity of the assessment procedure are important. In general, an assessment device is *reliable* to the extent that it yields a consistent outcome (score, tally) as long as the target behavior does not change. Reliability is often established by the test–retest method, in which a number of individuals are tested with the same instrument on two successive occasions and the mathematical relation (i.e., correlation) between the sets of scores is calculated. This relation is expressed in terms of a correlation coefficient, which can range from 0.0 to 1.0; the higher the value, the more reliable the instrument. Standardized assessment instruments often provide information concerning reliability; as a rule of thumb, values of 0.9 or above are desirable.

A measurement procedure is *valid* to the extent that it measures what it purports to measure. Validity typically is not determined directly but is inferred on the basis of whether the instrument is (a) logically defensible, (b) similar in concept and outcome to other accepted measures of the same behavior, and (c) accepted by experts.

A *sensitive* measure is one that is capable of showing drug effects when they occur. Sensitivity ultimately is determined by empirical test, but it is clear that a measure can be sensitive only if it reflects the target behavior and is subject to change. The importance of valid, reliable, and sensitive assessment procedures will become clear if we consider a situation in which John's height and weight, not his behavior, are measured.

The use of an easily stretched rubber ruler to measure height is a good example of an unreliable instrument (Salvia & Ysseldyke, 1981). If John's height were measured several times in a 1-hour period by different adults using such a ruler, it is likely that the obtained values would vary considerably because the measured height depends not only on the distance from the floor to the top of John's head (which would not change much in an hour), but also on how strongly the ruler is stretched. The measurement system is unreliable to the extent that it yields different values with repeated assessments. Assume that, for reasons that need not concern us, John's height was measured 10 times in an hour and values of 36.7, 45, 37.2, 56.1, 29, 32.2, 37.4, 35, 31.1, and 40.6 inches were obtained. How tall is he? It's impossible to say with any confidence. One can only conclude that his height (as measured with a stretchable rubber ruler) is somewhere between 29 and 56.1 inches. The difference between these values is so great that the information is practically meaningless.

Reliability generally can be improved by ensuring that measures are taken in a consistent fashion. If a concerted effort were made always to stretch the ruler with the same force, 10 consecutive determinations of John's height might yield values of 36, 35.4, 35.9, 36.1, 35.8, 36.3, 35.9, 36, and 36.2 inches. These values tell us that John is about 36 inches tall. Although there is some variability across observations (as occurs with all measurement systems), it is probably small enough to be of no practical significance. For most uses in which height data are employed, for instance, buying clothes, a height of 35.4 inches (the least value in our set of 10 measurements) is not significantly different from one of 36.3 inches (the greatest value in our set of 10).

If the data are to be put to such uses, however, it is crucial that the inches measured with the rubber ruler are equivalent to those used by clothing manufacturers. In all likelihood, they would not be, for the distance between lines designating an inch on an easily elongated rubber ruler is not fixed but varies according to how hard the ruler is stretched. Therefore the rubber ruler (like any other unreliable or inaccurate assessment device) should be replaced by a better instrument, perhaps a rigid plastic ruler calibrated in standard inches. If used consistently to measure the distance from the floor to the top of John's head, a rigid ruler provides repeatable data and is therefore reliable. Moreover, because the dimension being assessed is height as it is usually conceived, the ruler is valid. It would not, of course, be a valid measure of weight. A number of workable strategies for quantifying weight can be envisioned, but no reasonable person argues that weight can be validly assessed with a ruler. Unfortunately, the validity of procedures used to quantify behavior can rarely be determined so easily.

Weight is validly assessed with a scale, but scales differ in many regards, including their sensitivity. For example, John's weight could be measured by either a bathroom scale or a truck scale. The former indicates weight rounded to the nearest 1 pound, the latter indicates weight rounded to the nearest 100 pounds. Both yield reliable measures, but the bathroom scale certainly provides a more sensitive measure of John's weight than the truck scale and is a more useful instrument for any conceivable application.

Let us return to the assessment of John's behavior. A large number of different tests, tasks, rating scales and direct observation procedures are used by researchers and clinicians to evaluate behavior problems, activity level, interactions with peers and adults, and academic, cognitive, and motor performance in hyperactive children (Ross & Ross, 1982; Werry, 1978; see also chapter 6). Techniques for assessing John's response to medication should be selected before treatment is initiated. Unfortunately, because they are not able to observe patients in the locations where their behaviors constitute a problem, physicians responsible for prescribing a psychotropic medication rarely collect the information required to evaluate its efficacy. John's physician in all likelihood does not observe the boy at home or at school even though these are the locations where his behaviors constitute a problem. To determine if methylphenidate is producing the desired effect, the physician must therefore rely on the observations of John's care-providers. If their observations accurately portray the level of occurrences in the situation of concern, they are said to be ecologically valid.

With many somatic diseases, ecological validity is not a problem, because the signs and symptoms of distress change little across situations and are detectable with tests of biological function or laboratory assays of tissue and fluids. Envision a woman with strep throat. Her primary problem is pain, which she experiences in the physician's office and everywhere else. Other significant indications of the disease, including swelling, inflammation, increased body temperature, and a proliferation of *Streptococcus pyogenes* bacteria, also are apparent wherever she goes. Because of this, evaluating a medication prescribed to deal with strep throat (perhaps penicillin) is relatively simple. The physician can through direct observation and conversation with the patient readily index the severity of the disease before and after penicillin is given and in that way determine its efficacy.

In contrast, John's symptoms and his response to methylphenidate are difficult to evaluate in the physician's office. The way he behaves depends critically on his environment; a short sample of behavior in the physician's office does not provide a clear picture of what he does elsewhere. Recognizing this, the physician should seek information (data) about John's functioning at home and at school. General strategies for collecting such data are discussed shortly.

Self-reports involve the patient verbally describing his or her condition. They can easily be obtained with patients who are verbal and compliant, and they enable a physician to gain information about past events and the patient's mood, thoughts, and overt behavior in the situation of clinical concern. Despite these advantages, self-reports are not especially compelling indices of drug response, for it is difficult to determine their reliability and validity and they are easily affected by nondrug variables. Nonetheless, what a person says about the problems for which medication is prescribed always merits attention and is in some cases of crucial importance. One could not, for example, easily assess the usefulness of a medication prescribed to treat an affective disorder unless the patient described his or her subjective state (mood) in the presence and absence of the drug. Unfortunately, some patients are unable to describe their own thoughts, feelings, and overt behaviors.

Evaluating unstructured self-reports requires considerable skill because they do not directly yield quantitative information. A depressed person may, for example, report "feeling better and doing more things" after treatment with imipramine (Tofranil), but this does not allow for a precise comparison of affect and activity before and after drug administration. Asking the patient to rate his or her mood, perhaps on a scale of 1 (most depressed) to 10 (least depressed), and to count the times each week she or he engages in certain kinds of activities (e.g., contacts friends, goes out, oversleeps, has trouble falling asleep) would help to quantify changes in behavior and might be a useful supplement to unstructured verbal comments. Having another person (e.g., a spouse) rate the patient's mood and collect data on these same behaviors would provide a check on the accuracy of the self-reports and generate information useful in its own right.

Self-reports are useful in the detection of adverse drug effects, and by alerting the patient to possible side effects may increase the probability of detection. It is especially difficult to detect side effects in patients without expressive language. As Greinier (1958) noted nearly two decades ago,

> Sensible adult patients will usually balk when a drug is causing symptoms, but the very young and the very old are forced to take drugs, can't complain or stop on toxic symptoms, may not even connect them with the drug. The mentally deficient of any size or age cannot protect themselves either, and they also merit special care to avoid toxic doses. (p. 349)

Global clinical impression is a common and easily accomplished method for evaluating psychotropic medications. In forming such an impression, the evaluator typically takes into account the patient's verbal behavior, nonverbal behavior, and general appearance, although procedures for evaluating these dimensions are not formalized. Global clinical impression of a person labeled as schizophrenic, for instance, depends in part on the extent to which the content of the patient's speech provides evidence of hallucinations, delusions, illogical thinking, and in-appropriate affect.

The utility of the method is somewhat limited because it is not al-ways apparent what aspects of a patient's symptoms or general behav-ior a clinician is evaluating or whether the evaluation is valid and reli-able. Moreover, unless the global impression is based on observations of behavior in the situation of clinical concern, its ecological validity is questionable. Finally, it is difficult to quantify degree of improvement when global clinical impression is used. The typical procedure is to rate the patient's behavior along a continuum ranging from much improved to much worsened, a crude system at best.

Despite these shortcomings, global clinical impression can play a significant role in the practical evaluation of psychotropic medications, especially when augmented by other, less subjective sources of infor-mation. Surely clinicians can detect significant changes in the trouble-some behaviors of their patients. Parents can also detect changes in the behavior of their children, teachers in that of their students, and spouses in that of their mates. When making global clinical ratings, one should always focus on the problem that led to the prescription of medication. For example, a drug intended to reduce self-injurious behavior in a mentally retarded adolescent is efficacious if, and only if, self-injurious behavior is significantly reduced when medication is administered. Other advantageous changes in behavior, such as an increase in attention or a reduction in self-stimulatory behavior, are serendipitous effects but in themselves do not verify the efficacy of treatment. They might, how-ever, enhance global impressions.

Direct observation of behavior involves someone actually watching the patient in the situation of clinical concern and recording the patient's behavior. This procedure requires the use of trained observers (who can be expensive to procure), and it can be difficult or impossible to arrange in some circumstances. Moreover, people sometimes behave differently when they are being observed, a problem called *reactivity of measurement*. This problem can be minimized by making observers as inconspicuous as possible.

Direct observation requires one to define carefully the target behav-iors, a significant point in its favor. In general, a good definition is objective, clear, and complete (Kazdin, 1982). A definition is *objective* if it specifies observable events, *clear* if it unambiguously describes the physical form of these events, and *complete* if it delineates the bound-aries for inclusion and noninclusion (i.e., enables the observer to know whether a response has or has not occurred). Consider one of John's problems in the classroom, a short attention span. Throughout the day John shifts rapidly from one activity to another and does not work for a sufficiently long period on assigned tasks. To quantify off-task behavior, we might have an observer watch John during a 30-minute academic period each morning and afternoon and record at the end of 10-second intervals whether he was off-task during that interval. Doing so requires a workable definition of "off-task behavior," such as "visual nonattention to one's materials for more than 2 sec, unless the student [is] either talking to the teacher (with permission) or had his hand raised above his head" (Iwata & Bailey, 1974, p. 568). This is an objective, clear, and complete operational definition of off-task behavior.

Simply put, the operational definition of a behavior is an exact specification of the way in which it is measured. The history of psychology has been marred by much fruitless debate concerning the meanings of terms such as attention, learning, and aggression. These debates have stemmed in large part from linguistic imprecision: People have shared a set of terms but have used them differently. Much confusion can be averted by the use of operational definitions that allow behavior to be scaled along real physical dimensions, such as magnitude, latency, duration, accuracy, frequency, and rate of occurrence.

Magnitude refers to the intensity of a behavior, for example, the force exerted in a manual task. *Latency* refers to the time elapsed between some environmental event and the onset of a response (e.g., light flash and pressing a button). The time between the onset and offset of a response defines *response duration*. *Accuracy* reflects the extent to which a response is appropriately controlled by environmental objects or events. Performance on an intelligence test is a measure of response accuracy in that the appropriateness of a given response is determined by the question that preceded it. *Frequency* refers to the absolute number of times that a response occurs, whereas *rate* denotes the number of occurrences per unit of time.

A response may constitute a problem by virtue of its topography (physical form) alone, or only when it occurs with inappropriate magnitude, accuracy, duration, or frequency. A cardinal rule in selecting an observation system is to be sure that the system adopted emphasizes those aspects of behavior that are change-worthy. Think about one of John's problem behaviors, aggression directed toward his sister. Although behavior labelled as aggressive can take many forms, let us assume that John's parents use the term to refer to recurring episodes in which the boy curses his sister, then (unless he is stopped) slaps and kicks her. Three dimensions of these episodes appear to be important: their frequency (or rate) of occurrence, their magnitude (intensity), and their duration. These dimensions interact to determine the likelihood of the girl's suffering harm and the general disruption of family harmony associated with John's aggressive behavior.

A moment's thought reveals that magnitude and duration are meaningful measures only if no one intervenes to alter John's behavior. If these aggressive episodes are serious enough to be a problem—and they are—adults must try to stop them as soon as possible. Here, magnitude and duration measures are neither practical nor useful. As this example indicates, practical and ethical considerations often influence the way in which target behaviors are quantified.

Many different observational systems are available, some of which are quite complex and allow for the simultaneous quantification of up to a dozen behaviors. For example, Marholin, Touchette and Stewart (1979) used direct observation to examine the effects of chlorpromazine (Thorazine) on several behaviors of mentally retarded adults. Among the responses measured were compliance to verbal requests, accuracy and rate of performance on workshop tasks, time on task, eye contact, talking to self, talking to others, standing, walking, being within three feet of others, being in bed, approaching others, and touching others. Quantifying all of these behaviors allowed for a broad-spectrum assessment of the behavioral effects of the drug.

Figure 3.1 shows how a single response (self-stimulatory behavior) would be quantified under each of six simple observational systems. This figure presents hypothetical data for frequency, rate, and percent-occurrence measures of aggressive behavior during one 10-minute observational period. Four different procedures for measuring percent occurrence are shown. Two are *time sampling* (or *interval recording*) procedures and two are *intermittent time sampling* (or *intermittent interval recording*) procedures. In the former type, the total observational period is divided into discrete intervals and the observer records whether or not the behavior appeared in each interval. In the latter, observation occurs in only a few intervals, typically selected at random from the total period of interest. With either observational system, *partial interval* or *whole interval* recording may be used. In partial interval recording, the observer scores (i.e., indicates that the target behavior occurred in) any interval in which the response definition was met, regardless of the duration of occurrence. In whole interval recording, an interval is scored only if the response definition was met throughout the interval. (There is no consensus as to the terms that should be used to describe specific observational procedures; the labels used here appear to capture the gist of the procedures to which they refer, but several alternatives have been offered.)

It is important to recognize that *different observational systems do not*

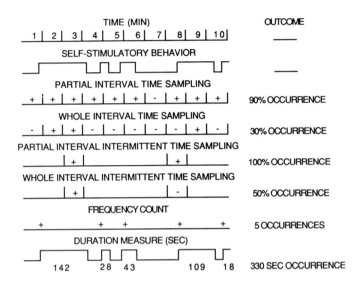

FIGURE 3.1. Hypothetical data showing how self-stimulatory behavior would be quantified using various strategies. Event records are used to indicate the occurrence of behavior; displacement of the line from the lower level indicates the behavior is occurring. In this example, the 10-min observational period is divided into 10 1-min observational periods for the time-sampling procedures, and two 1-min observational periods are arranged under the intermittent time-sampling procedures.

necessarily yield comparable outcomes. Therefore, the person responsible for designing observational systems should be aware of the range of procedures commonly employed and their characteristics. In general, observational systems that monitor behavior continuously (or as nearly so as possible) are to be preferred because the more often observation is arranged, the greater the likelihood that the findings reflect the general level of occurrence of target behaviors. Moreover, monitoring systems should provide information about all the aspects of the patient's behavior that the medication is prescribed to change. Simply determining whether methylphenidate reduced the frequency of John's aggressive episodes is not adequate. One must also examine the effects of the drug on other target behaviors that reflect attention, restlessness, and impulsivity. Provision also should be made to detect possible adverse behavioral and physiological actions of methylphenidate, which may require the use of data collection procedures other than direct observation.

Although direct observation is useful for quantifying behaviors not easily indexed in other ways, one cannot automatically assume that its findings accurately reflect the behavior of concern. Folklore suggests that lay observations are an imperfect reflection of actual happenings, and a sizeable body of information indicates that allegedly scientific observations sometimes provide an inaccurate description of phenomena. Among the variables demonstrated to influence reported observations are the observer's motivation and expectations, the observational procedures, and the characteristics of the behavior being monitored.

Researchers who use direct observation to quantify human behavior follow certain conventions intended to increase the quality of their data. They nearly always calculate interobserver agreement, which specifies the degree of correspondence obtained between the data recorded by two independent observers. A high degree of interobserver agreement indicates that observations are in one sense reliable and also shows that the response definition is a workable one. Interobserver agreement can be calculated in many ways (see Page & Iwata, 1986). One procedure commonly employed with interval recording is shown in Figure 3.2.

Researchers also characteristically employ "blind" observers (individuals not aware of the treatment conditions in effect) and make audiovisual tapes of the subject's behavior to check the accuracy of recorded data. Although it is not always possible to use such care in

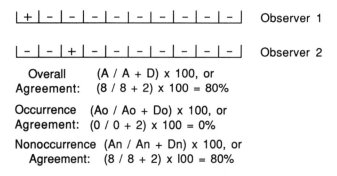

FIGURE 3.2. Hypothetical data recorded by each of two observers who independently scored the behavior of the same patient. A "+" in an observational interval indicates that the behavior occurred; a "−" indicates that it did not occur. Also shown are calculations for determining percentage measures of overall interobserver agreement. In the equations, A represents intervals in which the observers agreed in their ratings and D represents intervals in which the observers disagreed. An o after either A or D indicates that only intervals in which at least one observer recorded a + are being considered, whereas an n indicates that only intervals in which at least one observer recorded a − are being considered. Note that overall and nonoccurrence agreement measures are relatively high (80%) in this example, but occurrence agreement is low (0%). Although overall agreement and nonoccurrence agreement are identical in this example, this is not necessarily the case.

the practical evaluation of medication, many situations will allow for the employment of "blind" observers and the calculation of interobserver agreement.

Automated recording devices make it simple to quantify certain behaviors. For instance, the amount of time that John remains seated during a teaching session can be measured by affixing a contact-operated switch to the seat of his chair and having this switch, when operated, activate a running time meter. Unfortunately, automated recording devices are often complicated and expensive, and many significant behaviors cannot be directly quantified by machines.

Audio and video recording devices can be used to make lasting records of behavior, which can be used to check the accuracy of data recorded by observers. Moreover, these lasting records allow one to score responses when convenient. In those situations where audiovisual recording can be readily accomplished (e.g., in many schools), it can play a valuable role in the practical evaluation of psychotropic medications.

Physiological assessment involves directly monitoring bodily function. This is often done with automated equipment, which increases overall objectivity and accuracy of measurement. Physiological measures are important for assessing side effects of some drugs. For example, the antiepileptic drug carbamazepine (Tegretol) sometimes depresses bone marrow function and produces a variety of serious hematological disorders. Although rare, these reactions are serious to the point of being life-threatening and may be irreversible. It is generally recommended, therefore, that individuals who take carbamazepine have routine blood tests.

Physiological measures are sometimes used to measure anxiety and other clinical states. It is revealing that when physiological, motoric, and self-report data are collected simultaneously to quantify a particular clinical problem (e.g., a phobia), treatment often fails to produce equivalent effects across the three dimensions (Hersen & Barlow, 1976). As Paul (1967) contended, "While multiple measures of outcome are necessary, the dependent variable in any outcome evaluation must be . . . change in the disturbing behavior which brought the client to treatment" (p. 112).

Analog methods involve assessing behavior outside the environment in which it is of clinical concern. Analog methods simulate the situation of concern in a way that allows behavior to be easily and safely monitored. For example, a driving simulator requires the operator to engage in behaviors similar to those needed to drive an automobile on the highway. Measuring how well these behaviors are performed in the presence and absence of a drug allows one to assess whether the medication is likely to reduce the ability to operate a motor vehicle safely.

One important potential problem with analog methods is low ecological validity: The effects observed in the analog situation may not accurately reflect a patient's response to medication in the actual situation. When they do, analog methods can be quite useful in research and clinical applications. For example, laboratory measures of learning, short-term memory, reaction time, sustained attention, and motor performance are available and can be fruitfully employed to analyze response to medication (see Gadow, 1986a; Poling, 1986). Unfortunately, many of these procedures require rather elaborate material and a good deal of methodological sophistication. This limits their applications for practically evaluating medication effects outside research settings.

Checklists and rating scales are widely used in assessing medication effects. For example, the Teachers Rating Scale, of which there are several versions (e.g., Conners, 1969, 1973), and the Abbreviated Teacher Rating Scale (Conners, 1973) are frequently used in quantifying symptoms of hyperactivity and in evaluating drug effects thereon. The Hamilton Rating Scale (Hamilton, 1967), used to index severity of depression, and the Aberrant Behavior Checklist (Aman, Singh, Steward, & Field, 1985), designed specifically for evaluating psychotropic drug effects in mentally retarded people, are examples of other commonly employed instruments. Checklists and rating scales are easy and inexpensive to use, which is a real asset. The critical requirement when these devices are employed is correspondence between raters' evaluations and important aspects of the patient's behavior. When it is clear that checklists or rating scales provide accurate measures of target behaviors, they are simple and cost-effective assessment devices.

Rating scales can be very sensitive to drug effects, as indicated by the comments of Sleator and Sprague (1978) concerning the use of teacher rating scales in evaluating stimulant medications:

> Remarkable sensitivity to drug effects on the part of the teacher has been replicated regularly in our laboratory. No other clinical measure even approaches this sensitivity [and] we recommend strongly that monitoring of drug effects must include reports from the teacher if the physician hopes to effectively treat school children with learning and/or behavior disorders. He must be in active communication with the child's teacher. The physician would not consider treating anemias, for example, without repeated laboratory tests. For the child with learning problems the teacher is the physician's laboratory. (p. 579)

Rating scales and checklists may detect changes in behavior other than those that medication is intended to produce. Table 3.1 lists a number of rating scales designed specifically to assess side effects of medication. Scales for rating tardive dyskinesia (involuntary motor activity produced by neuroleptic drugs) are considered in chapter 4. One

Table 3.1. Selected Side-Effect Rating Scales

Scale*	Source	Side Effects Evaluated
Abnormal Involuntary Movement Scale (A.I.M.S.)	Borison (1985)	Acute extrapyramidal side effects (akathisia, dystonia, pseudo-parkinsonism)
Dosage Record and Treatment Emergent Symptom Scale (DOTES)	NIMH† (1985a)	General side effects
Monitoring of Side-Effects System (MOSES)	Kalachnik (1985)	General side effects
Neurological rating scale	Simpson & Angus (1970)	Acute extrapyramidal side effects
Parent's interval rating scales for side effects (also scales for physicians asking children)	Gofman (1972–1973)	General side effects
Systematic Assessment for Treatment Emergent Effects (SAFTEE)	NIMH (1986)	General side effects
Subjective Treatment Emergent Symptoms Scale (STRESS)	NIMH (1985b)	General side effects
Systematic toxicity rating scale, neurotoxicity rating scale, seizure type and frequency rating	Cramer et al. (1983)	Antiepileptic effects and general side effects
Withdrawal Emergent Symptoms Checklist (WESC)	Engelhardt (1974)	General drug-withdrawal side effects

*For scales with an accepted acronym, it is listed in parentheses.
†NIMH = National Institutes of Mental Health
From "Medication Monitoring Procedures" (p. 243) by John E. Kalachnik, 1988, in K. D. Gadow & A. Poling, *Pharmacotherapy and Mental Retardation*, 1988, San Diego, College-Hill Press. Copyright 1988 by College-Hill Press. Reproduced by permission.

scale for rating general side effects, termed the Monitoring of Side-Effects System (MOSES), is presented in Appendix B.

Standardized personality and intelligence tests appear to be of relatively little value in evaluating psychotropic medication, for they are (a) not designed for this purpose, (b) an indirect measure of the behaviors medication is intended to improve, and (c) often of limited sensitivity. However, of the wide range of standardized tests available, some are occasionally useful in drug evaluations, especially when used in combination with other measures. When such tests are used, one must be certain that they are valid and reliable for the population of concern. Many intelligence tests, for example, are of unknown validity and reliability when administered to mentally retarded people.

Special programs in which some patients participate provide data that can be quite useful in evaluating psychotropic medication. The academic performance of students, for instance, is regularly evaluated and can be used to index drug effects. Some patients who live in controlled environments (e.g., psychiatric hospitals, residential facilities) receive treatment under token economy systems that require the collection of data concerning a number of important behaviors. These data can be used in the treatment evaluation. Other patients work in situations where their vocational performance is monitored (e.g., sheltered workshops) and can be compared on and off medication. Care must be taken, however, to ensure that the information actually relates to the behavior problems that the psychotropic drug is prescribed to treat. It is surprisingly easy to emphasize aspects of a patients' behavior that are easy to quantify, or are being quantified prior to medication, without considering whether or not these aspects are change-worthy and therefore important.

In circumstances where psychotropic drugs are regularly evaluated (e.g., state hospitals for the mentally ill), it is useful to set in place general procedures that document the overall behavior of each patient. These procedures, combined with specific assessments designed to quantify the responses that are especially important for individual clients, provide a useful and cost-effective method for profiling the effects of medication.

EVALUATING THE RESPONSE TO MEDICATION

The steps involved in selecting and evaluating a psychotropic drug, outlined in Figure 3.3, are simple in principle. The patient is initially assessed, a general drug class and a specific agent are determined, a dosing regimen is selected, and the medication is administered. Data concerning therapeutic and side effects are collected before and during treatment and evaluated by the physician (ideally in consultation with other caregivers and the patient). Depending on outcome, a decision is made to continue treatment as initiated, to alter dosage, to change to another medication, or to terminate pharmacological manipulations.

If all goes well, the initial medication regimen or a subsequent treatment solves the behavior problem. In other words, the change in behavior observed when medication is administered is clinically significant. A *clinically significant* change in behavior is one that actually benefits the patient. An *experimentally significant* change in behavior, in contrast, is one that can be attributed with confidence to the intervention, re-

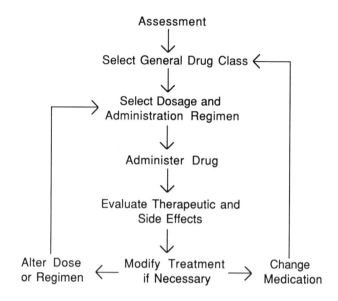

FIGURE 3.3. Simplified sequence of the steps involved in the pharmacological management of a behavior problem. The steps are described in the text.

gardless of its magnitude or benefit to the patient. Clinical significance can be evaluated in three general ways:

1. By having those who sought treatment for the behavior problem evaluate the success of the intervention. John's behavior caused a problem for his parents and his teacher when the boy was not receiving medication. If methylphenidate produces the desired effect, they should consider his behavior as significantly improved (i.e., no longer a problem or at least more manageable) when the drug is administered. The difficulty with this approach is that it relies on global impressions, which may be inaccurate or reflect dimensions of behavior other than those the medication is intended to alter.

2. By comparing levels of behavior during treatment with criterion levels set before treatment. These criterion levels (treatment objectives) constitute the solution of the behavior problem for which medication is prescribed. Those responsible for seeking treatment, the patient (insofar as possible), and the physician should interact to set treatment goals specified in objective, quantitative terms prior to the onset of treatment. The advantages of this approach are that it is not subjective and it focuses attention on the precise goals of treatment. Reaching a consensus concerning appropriate treatment objectives can, however, be difficult. Moreover, placing undue emphasis on a priori criteria for success can lead to narrow and unwise decisions concerning the efficacy of a medication, especially if those criteria are unrealistic.

3. By comparing the performance of the person undergoing treatment with that of similar individuals who do not manifest the same behavioral problem. If, for example, John engages in no more off-task behavior when receiving methylphenidate than his classmates, there is no reason to consider this aspect of his behavior as a problem. It is difficult in some cases to determine with whom a treated patient should be compared, however; and even if an appropriate comparison group is determined, it may be it difficult to quantify their behavior.

Evaluation of clinical significance always requires consideration of deleterious side effects as well as desired alterations in behavior, which is a risk–benefit analysis. Whether any undesirable action of a psychotropic medication is offset by treatment gains can be adequately determined only by comparison with the relative costs and benefits of alternative treatments. In view of the potentially restrictive (harmful) nature of psychotropic drug treatments, Sprague and Baxley (1978) have recommended that they always be compared with some other intervention, preferably the best alternative available.

Side effects as well as therapeutic effects must be considered in comparing diverse treatments. Detecting adverse drug reactions can be difficult, especially when they are insidious (emerging only with long exposure), or appear only when medication is withdrawn. Side effects of other treatments may also escape easy detection. Even when the side and therapeutic effects of two dissimilar treatments are known, ascertaining the better treatment may be difficult because doing so usually entails an "apples and oranges" comparison. The side effects of different treatments are rarely similar in kind or in magnitude, and therapeutic effects, too, may differ in subtle ways.

In many cases, the patient and physician can agree on the preferred treatment after discussing the probable effects of each alternative. Sometimes, however, the patient's condition does not allow him or her to participate meaningfully in treatment selection. In such cases, it is important that those making the choice keep the patient's best interest in mind. Caregivers are remiss in selecting treatments on the basis of cost, ease of implementation, or convenience of staff.

ATTRIBUTING BEHAVIOR CHANGE TO MEDICATION

Whether a drug improves, worsens, or has no effect on target behaviors can be determined only by comparing a patient's performance when drug is and is not given. At its simplest, the comparison involves initially recording behavior during a no-drug (baseline) condition, then administering drug and continuing to monitor behavior during this phase. In the shorthand used to describe experiments, this is an A-B design. (You will recall that practical drug evaluations are in a real sense experiments, even though they are usually not conducted by scientists.)

The primary advantage of an A-B design is the ease with which it is arranged. It is common practice in medicine first to assess and quantify a client's problem, then to implement a treatment designed to alleviate it. Assessment continues while treatment is in effect, and a comparison of measures taken before and during treatment determines the worth of the intervention. This is similar to what a person with a headache does when she or he takes a single 5-grain aspirin tablet and attempts to determine whether it alleviates pain. The strategy is compelling enough to convince most of us whether aspirin is of value in dealing with our headaches, but conservative sufferers might wish to test the drug a number of times before reaching a firm conclusion. Of course, if one wanted to describe aspirin's effects to a friend, some method would have to be devised for quantifying the magnitude of the perceived pain at various times before and after it was taken. Even if this were done and the severity of the headache progressively declined from the time the tablet was swallowed, a skeptic could argue that this did not prove anything about the drug's action: Pain might simply have begun to diminish at the time the drug was taken, whether or not aspirin was ingested. Thus, the skeptic can proclaim little faith in the analgesic action of aspirin, although the headachy individual staunchly advocates the drug.

The foregoing example calls to attention four important points concerning drug evaluations. First, a drug evaluation that convinces one person of the efficacy of a medication may not convince someone else. Clinical drug evaluation can be very conservative, adhering to the many dictates of scientific analysis, or more liberal, even haphazard. Second, as noted earlier, a drug cannot be adequately evaluated unless the behaviors of interest are appropriately measured. Third, when an observed relation between drug treatment and a particular outcome can be repeated, faith grows that the relation is real. Fourth, some drug evaluations are such that observed changes in behavior cannot be attributed with confidence to drug administration. Drug evaluations that employ an A-B design fall into this category.

Because of its logical structure, the A-B design can provide only weak and equivocal confirmation of a drug's behavioral effects. When this design is used, one can never be sure that a change in behavior that occurs coincidentally with intervention is not the result of another, unknown variable (*extraneous variable*) that became operative coincidentally with drug administration. Consider the physical assaults that John made on his sister. These episodes are appropriately defined and recorded and, during the 2 weeks prior to the administration of methylphenidate, occurred on average 6 times per day with a range across days of 3 to 14 episodes. On average, less than 1 assault per day occurred during the first 2 weeks that drug was given; the range across days was 0 to 2 episodes. Given these data, it can be safely asserted that the problem behavior occurred less often when John was medicated. It is by no means obvious, however, that the medication actually was responsible for the observed, and quite real, improvement.

Assume that John was perfectly healthy at the start of the assessment period. After 2 weeks, he became ill with a viral infection. This illness generally reduced his activity, including physical assaults, and was responsible for the lessened frequency of the target behavior when drug was administered. In this example, the extraneous variable of illness could be easily detected by the boy's parents. Other extraneous variables that can produce effects like those desired of treatment, however, are difficult to detect. The A-B design does not adequately control for extraneous variables and for that reason is of little value to researchers. Nonetheless, if target behaviors have been relatively stable for a considerable period prior to treatment and clearly change in the desired direction and to the desired extent when medication is administered, this at least suggests that treatment is effective.

A more persuasive test of efficacy than that afforded by the A-B design can be arranged by terminating drug administration (or decreasing dosage) for a short period of time and determining whether target behaviors return to pretreatment levels. Adding a second no-drug (or baseline) phase to the A-B makes it an A-B-A experimental design, the logic of which is simple and direct: If the target behaviors improve appreciably relative to predrug levels when medication is administered and return to at- or near-baseline levels when drug is withdrawn, there is good reason to believe that the observed changes in the target behavior are actual effects of medication. Figure 3.4 shows hypothetical data for John's hyperactive behaviors as rated by his teacher, using the Abbreviated Teacher Rating Scale (Conners, 1973). This scale (see chapter 6) measures several behaviors associated with hyperactivity and yields a score ranging from 0 (no hyperactivity) to 30 (extreme hyperactivity).

As shown in Figure 3.4, the teacher rated John's behavior once a week (every Thursday). During the first 8 weeks, no medication was given. Methylphenidate (15 mg morning and noon) was administered during the next 12 weeks and was withdrawn during the final 6 weeks of the evaluation. Results are straightforward. Ratings ranged from 14 to 23 during the initial baseline period, from 5 to 11 when methylphenidate was given, and from 13 to 22 when medication was withdrawn.

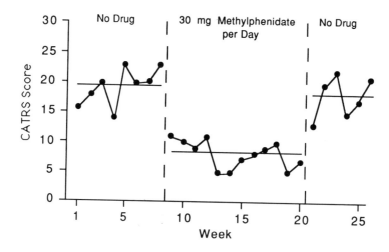

FIGURE 3.4. Hypothetical data for John's hyperactive behaviors as rated by his teacher using the Conners' Abbreviated Teacher Rating Scale (CATRS). The teacher rated his behavior each Thursday under conditions where a daily dose of 30 mg methylphenidate was (weeks 9 through 20) and was not (weeks 1 through 8 and 21 through 26) administered. Horizontal lines through the data points represents the average score for a condition. Based on the information shown in this figure, it appears that John benefitted significantly from treatment with methylphenidate.

Although these data alone are not sufficient to document the efficacy of treatment (at minimum, one would also need to ascertain whether any serious adverse reactions occurred), they do strongly suggest that methylphenidate substantially reduced hyperactive behaviors as indexed by the rating scale. This finding provides a reasonable justification for the treatment.

The A-B-A design (and similar configurations, such as the A-B-A-B or B-A-B) provide more convincing tests of efficacy than the A-B. The primary problem with the A-B-A design is that it may not be practically or ethically acceptable to stop administering a medication that appears to be producing clinically significant effects. John's teacher and parents, for example, may be understandably pleased that his behavior improved when methylphenidate was administered and see no need to terminate treatment just to demonstrate further the efficacy of methylphenidate. But it is generally accepted that no person should receive behavior-change medications for long, uninterrupted intervals. Drug-free (or reduced-dosage) periods are an accepted part of treatment with most psychotropic medications. They are a necessary part of clinical evaluation, not just to demonstrate efficacy but also to detect some patients who initially improve with medication but do not show deterioration when it is withdrawn. The frequency with which drug-free periods should be arranged, their duration, and the schedule of medication withdrawal vary according to particulars of the individual case, including the medication involved, the severity of the behavioral problem, and the apparent response to treatment.

It is important to recognize that abrupt termination of treatment with many kinds of drugs (including antianxiety agents, antidepressants, antipsychotics, and antiepileptics) can precipitate withdrawal reactions, especially when a patient has received moderate to high doses for a long time. "Care providers must therefore be careful not to overreact and confuse such reactions with the need to reinstate medication. To avoid the occurrence of withdrawal reactions, gradual dosage reductions are widely recommended" (Kalachnik, 1988, p. 254). What constitutes a gradual reduction varies with different drug classes. Taking neuroleptics as an example, Kalachnik notes that reported reduction procedures have involved 10% decreases every 3 to 7 days, 25% to 35% of the total dose per month, 25% to 33% of the total dose per month, 10% to 25% of the total dose per month, and 10% to 15% of the total dose every 2 or 3 months.

Regardless of the evaluative procedures, one can never be absolutely certain that observed changes in behavior are a direct result of medication. With, for example, an A-B-A design, it is possible that some extraneous variable begins to act upon the patient when medication is introduced, remains operative throughout the course of treatment, and then ceases when treatment is terminated. Recall the example of how John's viral infection may have reduced his aggressive episodes. If methylphenidate were introduced at the time the infection began, the effects of the infection might have been wrongly attributed to the drug with an A-B-A design if the illness ended at the same time medication was withdrawn. Unless an extraneous variable is actually associated with treatment, the odds that it will begin and end coincidentally with the medication regimen is low, but never nonexistent.

PLACEBO EFFECTS

A set of complex and interactive extraneous variables combine to produce what are termed *placebo effects*. The term placebo comes from a Latin root meaning "I shall please." A definition of placebo widely accepted today was proposed by Shapiro and Morris (1978). According to them, a *placebo* is "any therapy or component of therapy that is deliberately used for its nonspecific psychological or psychophysiological effect, or that is used for its presumed specific effect, but is without specific activity for the condition being treated" (p. 371).

It is widely recognized in medicine that simply exposing a patient to a placebo may produce real and clinically significant physiological and behavioral changes (e.g., Gadow, White & Ferguson, 1986a, 1986b; White, Tursky & Schwartz, 1985). These reactions can be favorable or unfavorable. The former are termed positive placebo effects, the latter negative placebo effects. As placebo effects occur with active medications as well as with inert placebos, the overall effect of a psychotropic medication is the sum of the direct pharmacological effects of the drug and any placebo effects it produces.

Conventional explanations of placebo effects are mentalistic. For example, according to Blaschke, Nies and Mamelok (1985), "Placebo effects result from the physician-patient relationship, the significance of the therapeutic effect to the patient, and the mental 'set' imparted by the therapeutic setting and by the physician" (p. 55). From a behavioral perspective, placebo effects are learned responses that depend in large part on the patient's history with respect to the medication administered and similar drugs and the rules he or she is given concerning the probable effects of treatment (see Poling, 1986). Regardless of how placebo effects are explained, they are important in evaluating the efficacy of a medication.

In research settings it is standard practice to employ placebo controls. In a *placebo-controlled* study, target behaviors are compared during conditions in which an active drug and a placebo preparation identical to the active drug in appearance are administered. Placebo-controlled conditions are used to prevent nonpharmacological variables that are inextricably associated with the act of giving medication (of which there are many) from obscuring the assessment of drug effects. The actions of such variables can be detected by including an experimental condition in which neither drug nor placebo is given.

Because it would make little sense to employ placebo controls if participants were told whether placebo or active drug was administered, *double-blind conditions* are also employed in research settings. When such conditions are in effect, neither patients nor caregivers (including those who evaluate the behavior of patients) are informed as to whether or not the pill being administered is a placebo or a "real" drug. Used together, double-blind procedures and placebo controls help to avoid confusing nonpharmacological with pharmacological effects of treatment.

Despite their overwhelming importance in clinical drug research, double-blind and placebo-controlled conditions play a limited role in everyday evaluation of psychotropic medication. The practical problems inherent in arranging double-blind and placebo-controlled conditions (e.g., formulating a placebo that resembles active medication and orchestrating human interactions to administer appropriate treatment, although neither the patient nor the caregivers know what it is) make them unappealing in many circumstances.

How, if placebo-controlled and double-blind conditions are not employed, can one be certain that what appear to be direct pharmacological effects of the medication are not actually placebo effects? In truth, one can never be absolutely sure. In many cases, however, interactions between the patient and the physician (or other caregivers) prior to the administration of medication serve much the same role as an actual placebo condition. That is, they evoke placebo responses. As Blaschke et al. (1985) contended with respect to the routine practice of medicine, "Although the inert medication may be an effective vehicle for a placebo effect, the physician-patient relationship is generally preferable" (p. 55).

When double-blind conditions cannot be arranged, care must be taken to ensure that target behaviors are measured in objective fashion and that the patient is, save with respect to whether or not medication is administered, always treated in comparable fashion. One reason that double-blind conditions are used in research settings is to reduce the possibility of placebo responses. Another is to prevent caregivers from treating a patient differently (which might result in a special kind of placebo effect), or rating his or her behavior in different ways, as a function of the presence or absence of medication. Consider a scenario in which John's teacher believed that methylphenidate was a useless and potentially harmful treatment for the boy. The teacher's ratings of his behavior might reflect this and be *biased* in the sense that a given pattern of responding would be rated as more of a problem when methylphenidate was administered than when it was withheld. The teacher might also treat the boy differently when drug was and was not given, perhaps acting in ways that led to more occurrences of undesirable behavior during the drug condition. In either case, the evaluation of methylphenidate would not be a fair and unbiased one. Fortunately, the likelihood of observer bias strongly affecting the outcome of a drug evaluation appears to be relatively low. Nevertheless, an interested party who strongly favors or abhors a particular medication should not play the primary role in its evaluation. In fact, it is generally unwise to have any one person solely responsible for collecting data used in evaluating a medication or for evaluating the clinical significance of those data.

PATIENT COMPLIANCE

Even though the clinical benefit derived from a medication is likely to be reduced unless it is administered at the proper time and dosage, patients and caregivers often fail to follow the physician's instructions.

Patient noncompliance may involve omission of scheduled doses, administration of inappropriate doses, or premature termination of drug therapy. A number of variables influence the likelihood of noncompliance, including the kind of medication involved and its efficacy, the treatment environment, the presenting disorder, and the degree to which the importance of compliance is stressed by the physician (Haynes, Taylor & Sackett, 1979; Moore & Klonoff, 1986). Noncompliance is especially likely when chronic (protracted) exposure to medication is required.

Some patients are not personally responsible for taking their medication. Instead, they take the drug at the time and dosage arranged by caregivers. Although this might appear to avert the problem of noncompliance, it does not do so entirely, for some patients become quite adept at appearing to swallow medication that is actually held under the tongue and later expelled. Others regurgitate their medication. Moreover, instructing professional staff or family members in the proper administration of medication does not prevent their making errors or instituting well-intentioned but ill-informed dosage adjustments. A common form of patient-initiated dosage adjustment involves titrating dosage according to subjective state: The patient feels good and takes little or no medication or feels bad and takes more than the prescribed dose. This practice has little to recommend it. In general, adjustments in dosage or other aspects of the treatment regimen should be made only after consultation with the physician who prescribed the drug. Responses to psychotropic medication are often complex and time-dependent and may require specialized medical training to interpret properly. Tricyclic antidepressants, for example, often produce clinically significant mood alterations only after prolonged (i.e., 2 to 4 weeks) exposure. Unless a patient is aware of this, he or she might despair after taking such a drug for a week or two and increase (or otherwise change) the dose, which could be unfortunate. Although the patient has every right to be involved in decisions concerning his or her treatment, patient-initiated changes in medication that do not correspond to accepted medical practice make it difficult to evaluate efficacy and can harm the patient. As Moore and Klonoff (1986) point out:

> When medication is not taken as instructed, the clinician might attribute the lack of improvement to the failure of the prescribed drug. In an effort to remediate this, he or she might increase the dosage or administer a new drug. Thus, patients who do not comply are at risk to receive higher doses than their condition warrants, or a different drug that may produce troublesome side effects. In fact, a patient's condition could be exacerbated by a change in prescription that erroneously resulted from undetected noncompliance. (p. 223)

It is clear in view of these considerations that a concerted effort must be made to ensure that patients take medication at the times and dosages prescribed by their physician.

Determining whether they have done so can be difficult. The most direct methods for determining whether medication has been ingested are urine and serum assays. Physician's opinions, self-reports, and objective measures (e.g., pill counts by spouses) can also be used. Each of these measures has attendant strengths and weaknesses. The one best used depends upon the patient, the medication, and the setting in which treatment is being evaluated. Moore and Klonoff (1986) and Sleator (1985) provide detailed coverages of noncompliance and its assessment and management.

Although patient-initiated changes in drug regimen are rarely advisable, dosage adjustments by the physician routinely occur as a part of treatment. The manner in which dosage is adjusted depends on the disorder being treated, the medication involved, and the patient's response to the medication. As noted in chapter 2, it is common practice to begin treatment with a relatively low dose, then to titrate dosage as necessary. In general, the appearance of significant side effects dictates dose reduction, whereas a failure to produce the desired alterations in behavior indicates that dosage be increased sequentially until (a) the desired effect occurs, (b) significant side effects (including behavioral toxicity) appear, or (c) the maximal suggested dosage is reached. When chronic treatment is required to control behavior, a maintenance dose considerable lower than that required for initial behavior control is sometimes effective. This possibility can be evaluated by systematically reducing dosage until behavior deteriorates. In some cases (as discussed with respect to drug-free periods), this does not occur even when medication is completely withdrawn. In others, however, reduction of dosage below some threshold level results in behavioral deterioration, whereupon return to the prior dose is prudent.

Evaluating the effects of dosage adjustment is straightforward: One compares levels of the target behaviors (and untoward reactions) at the various doses of interest. The optimal dose is as a rule the lowest one that adequately controls target behaviors. This dose is termed the *minimal effective dose* and, as Kalachnik (1988) notes, "Almost without exception, clinicians and psychopharmacologists stress the use of the least amount of medication" (p. 254). Systematic procedures for establishing the minimal effective dose for individual patients have been developed and are available to the general public (e.g., Fielding, Murphy, Reagan and Peterson, 1980).

The minimal effective dose for a particular patient may change across time as a function of changes in his or her health or environment or of the concurrent administration of other medications. In view of this, evaluation of efficacy must continue for as long as the patient undergoes treatment.

CONCLUDING COMMENT

To determine whether a pharmacological intervention is successful in treating a behavior disorder, three questions must be answered: (1) What were the desired effects of the medication? (2) Were those effects obtained? (3) Were there any significant adverse reactions? Easy questions to ask, but not so easy to answer. Inadequate documentation of patients' response to treatment has been a recurrent problem in psychopharmacological research, and it is undoubtedly at least as difficult to evaluate drug effects in everyday clinical practice as in a research setting. But difficulty does not equal impossibility, and it is possible for other caregivers to work with physicians to ensure that patients are monitored in ways that allow both therapeutic and adverse reactions to be detected. Unless this is done, effective drug therapy for behavior disorders is unlikely.

Chapter 4

Neuroleptics

The neuroleptics are among the most commonly prescribed psychoactive agents, particularly in residential and hospital facilities for mentally retarded people, emotionally disturbed children and adolescents, psychiatric patients, and the elderly. In fact, hundreds of millions of children, adolescents, and adults have been treated with these medications worldwide since their introduction to modern medicine in the 1950s. Neuroleptics are generally safe and effective when used appropriately, rarely fatal (even upon consumption of extremely large doses as in suicide attempts), and therapeutically beneficial for a variety of mood, thought, and behavior disorders. Nevertheless, for some patients, they are completely ineffective, exacerbate symptoms, seriously impair adaptive behavior, produce somatic discomfort, or induce tormenting neurological syndromes. For these reasons, neuroleptic treatment is generally considered appropriate only for individuals whose symptoms are severe enough to justify the associated risks. When alternative agents of comparable efficacy and reduced toxicity are available, they are generally preferred.

The neuroleptics are categorized into several groups according to chemical structure: phenothiazines, butyrophenones, thioxanthenes, dihydroindolones, dibenzoxazepines, and diphenylbutylpiperidines. Table 4.1 lists the neuroleptics in each category that are approved for use in the United States. New neuroleptics are continually being discovered and marketed (more products are available in Europe); over the years, others have been withdrawn from distribution because of limited efficacy, unacceptable toxicity, or lack of commercial appeal.

As the phenothiazines are the most widely used neuroleptics, they are the primary focus of the following discussion. Although there are some marked differences in the prevalence of certain adverse drug re-

Table 4.1. Neuroleptic Drugs Marketed in the United States

Generic Name	Trade Name
PHENOTHIAZINES	
Aliphatic	
chlorpromazine	Thorazine
triflupromazine	Vesprin
Piperidine	
piperacetazine	Quide
mesoridazine	Serentil
thioridazine	Mellaril
Piperazine	
acetophenazine	Tindal
fluphenazine	Prolixin, Permitil
perphenazine	Trilafon
trifluoperazine	Stelazine
THIOXANTHENES	
chlorprothixene	Taractan
thiothixene	Navane
BUTYROPHENONE	
haloperidol	Haldol
DIHYDROINDOLONE	
molindone	Moban
DIBENZAZEPINE	
clozapine	Clozaril
DIBENZOXAZEPINE	
amoxapine	Asendin
loxapine	Loxitane
DIPHENYLBUTYLPIPERIDINE	
pimozide	Orap

Excluded are agents that are not commonly used at the present time for the management of psychiatric disorders (e.g., prochlorperazine, promazine).

actions, the neuroleptics are generally considered to produce similar therapeutic effects. They have proved to be effective in the suppression of some symptoms associated with autism, hyperactivity, mania, organic mental syndromes, schizophrenia, and Tourette syndrome. Baldessarini (1985) summarized the uses of neuroleptic drugs for the treatment of adolescent and adult psychiatric disorders as follows:

> The "target" symptoms for which the neuroleptic agents seem to be especially effective include tension, hyperactivity, combativeness, hostility, negativism, hallucinations, acute delusions, insomnia, poor self-care, excessive fasting, anorexia, and sometimes withdrawal and seclusiveness; less likely is improvement in insight, judgment, memory, and orientation. The most favorable prognosis is for patients with relatively acute illnesses of brief duration who had relatively healthy personalities prior to the illness. (p. 409)

Compounds similar in chemical structure to modern-day neuroleptics were first synthesized in the late 1800s. In the 1930s one of these compounds (promethazine) was found to have powerful antihistaminic and sedative effects. Promethazine (Phenergan) was tested in the 1940s for the treatment of agitation in psychiatric patients, but the results were not particularly encouraging. Because promethazine enhanced the effects of barbiturates, it was useful in clinical anesthesia. The search for more anesthesia-potentiating agents led to the synthesis of chlorpromazine (Thorazine, Largactil) by Charpentier in 1949–1950. The first attempts to use this new drug for the treatment of mental illness were conducted shortly thereafter.

In 1952 Delay and Deniker began their clinical trials with chlorpromazine. They are generally credited with introducing chlorpromazine into clinical psychiatry and discovering that it had specific antipsychotic properties. Reports of chlorpromazine's effectiveness for treating psychiatric patients and mentally retarded residents first appeared in the North American literature in 1954–1955; by December 1956, there were over 5,000 articles about chlorpromazine in the world literature (Wardell, Rubin & Ross, 1958). Since then, dozens of neuroleptic drugs have been developed and marketed. Some notable examples are thioridazine (Mellaril) and haloperidol (Haldol, Serenace), which were first approved for clinical use in the United States in 1959 and 1967, respectively.

The addition of chlorpromazine and other antipsychotic drugs to the list of available treatments in psychiatry had an extraordinary effect upon the lives of millions of mentally ill patients throughout the world. Prior to the 1950s, the most commonly prescribed psychoactive agents for the treatment of severe behavioral disturbance were bromides, barbiturates, and opiates (e.g., morphine), all of which had serious limitations (Lader, 1989). During the onset of treatment, some patients experienced transitory symptom exacerbation. Therapeutic doses often produced marked sedation to the point of deep sleep or even coma, and behavioral toxicity obscured the identification of target symptoms. Moreover, the termination of pharmacotherapy was complicated by the possible emergence of withdrawal syndromes and drug dependence. Chlorpromazine, however, was not for the most part, saddled with these problems, and neuroleptic medication rapidly became the treatment of first choice. These drugs had a profound impact on the hospital environment by directly decreasing physical assaults on staff and destruction of property and by indirectly reducing time spent in restraints and seclusion. Many patients were able to leave the psychiatric hospital, some to return home and resume work, others to receive outpatient care through community mental health agencies.

PHARMACOLOGY

The neuroleptics are highly lipid-soluble and pass readily through tissue membranes, but their absorption in the gastrointestinal tract is erratic and unpredictable, resulting in considerable between-patient differences in drug blood levels for the same oral dose (Friedel, 1984). Liquid concentrates of neuroleptic drugs are generally absorbed more rapidly than solids. Intramuscular injection can increase the rate of distribution to sites of action by 4 to 10 times and produces less variability in blood concentrations between patients.

Once in the bloodstream, neuroleptics become highly bound to plasma proteins. Approximate values in normal adults for several neuroleptics are as follows: chlorpromazine (95% to 98%), thioridazine (98%), and haloperidol (92%). The high rate of protein binding has clinical implications. Patients with abnormally high or low levels of plasma proteins (i.e., more or fewer binding sites) require higher and lower doses of neuroleptics, respectively. Other drugs that are also highly bound to plasma proteins can be a problem when administered in conjunction with a neuroleptic if both agents are competing for the same binding sites.

Neuroleptics are typically metabolized by liver enzymes into a variety of compounds, most of which are inactive. However, some of these biological transformations produce *active metabolites* (i.e., compounds capable of producing therapeutic and/or untoward effects). For example, thioridazine is transformed by liver enzymes into a number of metabolites, three of which appear in appreciable quantities in the blood: thioridazine-5-sulfoxide (inactive), sulforidazine (active), and mesoridazine (active). One of these metabolites, mesoridazine, is available in prescription form. Clinically, the important point with regard to neuroleptics and their metabolites is that blood assays of the parent compound may be of only limited value in generating treatment guidelines, monitoring therapeutic response, and understanding drug effects. Much research remains to be done in this area. Another aspect of drug metabolism that has clinical implications for chlorpromazine (and other phenothiazines) is *autoinduction*, the ability to increase the rate of its own metabolism. After a few weeks of treatment with the same dose, chlorpromazine blood levels drop appreciably as a result of this process.

The rate of drug metabolism varies with age. Infants and elderly people have a diminished capacity to metabolize and eliminate neuroleptics (compared with normal adults) and therefore should receive less medication on a mg/kg basis. Children, however, have a tendency to metabolize neuroleptics more quickly than adults and therefore may require higher doses (mg/kg) of medication.

The elimination of neuroleptics and their metabolites is performed primarily by the kidneys. Owing to their high affinity for tissue membranes, drug molecules and metabolites continue to be excreted for weeks following cessation of long-term treatment.

MECHANISM OF ACTION

Although the exact mechanism by which neuroleptics produce their antipsychotic effects is unknown, much theorizing has focused on their ability to interfere with the actions of the neurotransmitter dopamine, particularly in the mesocortical, limbic, and hypothalamic systems. The antidopaminergic actions of the neuroleptics also explain certain adverse drug reactions such as the extrapyramidal syndromes (discussed later in this chapter), which are thought to be produced by neurotransmitter dysfunction of the extrapyramidal tract, notably the basal ganglia, and increased prolactin secretion (regulated by the anterior pituitary), which may result in breast engorgement and *galactorrhea* (persistent flow of milk from the breasts). Neuroleptics also block the actions of neurotransmitters (acetylcholine and norepinephrine) released by peripheral motor neurons in the muscles and glands of the body, resulting in a wide array of side effects. The behavioral and physiological reactions that result from blocking the actions of acetylcholine are sometimes referred to as *anticholinergic* effects. Some examples of probable anticholinergic effects associated with chlorpromazine treatment are blurred vision, decreased gastric secretion and motility, and decreased sweating and salivation. Examples of chlorpromazine's norepinephrine blocking actions are *miosis* (contraction of the pupil) and *hypotension* (abnormally low blood pressure). Some neuroleptics also interfere with other neurotransmitters such as histamine, gamma-aminobutyric acid (GABA), and 5-hydroxytriptamine (5-HT), but the therapeutic implications of these actions (if any) are as yet unsubstantiated.

DOSE AND SCHEDULE

No single set of dosage guidelines covers all the disorders, age groups, patient populations, and desired therapeutic effects of neuroleptic drugs. For example, the dose of haloperidol prescribed for the control of tics in patients with Tourette syndrome is generally lower than the dose prescribed for hospitalized schizophrenics, and young autistic children are likely to receive higher doses than young Tourette syndrome patients. Menolascino et al. (1985) found that mentally retarded schizophrenics required lower doses of thiothixene (Navane) than nonretarded schizophrenics. In hyperactive children, Werry and Aman (1975) found that very low doses (0.025 mg/kg) of haloperidol enhanced attending behavior whereas higher doses did not. Given this situation, we present here general dosing guidelines for adults (see Table 4.2) and children (see Table 4.3) and note recommended doses for specific disorders in the section on efficacy.

There is a considerable range in the reported doses of neuroleptics across studies with children (Table 4.3). The average daily dose of thioridazine and chlorpromazine ranges from 75 to 150 mg per day. Some clinicians prescribe one large dose at night to prevent daytime drowsiness, whereas others divide the total amount into two or three doses during the day (Katz, Saraf, Gittelman-Klein & Klein, 1975; Winsberg & Yepes, 1978). Relative to body weight, the average dose is 3 to 6 mg/kg per day. The effective dose of haloperidol ranges from 2 to 5 mg per day, which is divided into three daily doses.

With regard to potency, the neuroleptics can be divided into two broad groups, the low-potency (usual mg dose is high) and the high-potency (usual mg dose is low) agents. By examining Table 4.2, one can see that fluphenazine (Prolixin, Permitil, Modicate), trifluoperazine (Stelazine), and haloperidol are in the high-potency group and that chlorpromazine and thioridazine are in the low-potency group. It can also be seen in Table 4.2 that the low-potency agents are generally much more sedating than the high-potency drugs and less likely to produce extrapyramidal reactions (discussed later in the chapter). The clinician can sometimes use this relationship to his or her advantage. For example, when confronted with a highly agitated patient in the emergency room, the sedative effects of chlorpromazine can be helpful. However, when managing long-term disorders, less sedating (sometimes referred to as "more stimulating") agents are clearly preferable.

Neuroleptic drug doses have been converted into a common metric sometimes referred to as *chlorpromazine equivalents* (Davis, 1976). In other words, the dose (in milligrams) of any neuroleptic drug can be converted to a comparable dose of chlorpromazine by using a simple ratio. In Table 4.2, for example, one can see that 1 mg of thiothixene is equal to approximately 25 mg of chlorpromazine.

There has been a general trend in recent years of ever-increasing preference for high-potency neuroleptics, which has resulted in an unfortunate problem. Physicians familiar with the high doses typically required for low-potency drugs have a tendency to prescribe higher than necessary doses of the high-potency neuroleptics (Baldessarini, Katz & Cotton, 1984). Subsequently, when patients are switched from

Table 4.2. Selected Neuroleptic Drugs: Adult Doses (schizophrenic patients) and Side Effects

Generic Name	Trade Name	Daily Oral Dose (mg)		Sedative Effects	Extrapyramidal Effects	Hypotensive Effects	Chlorpromazine Equivalence Ratio†
		Usual	Extreme*				
Phenothiazines							
acetophenazine	Tindal	60–120	20–600	++	++	+	1:4
chlorpromazine	Thorazine	300–800	25–2000	+++	++	++	1:1
fluphenazine	Prolixin, Permitil	1–20	0.5–30	+	+++	++	1:50
mesoridazine	Serentil	75–300	25–400	+++	+	++	1:2
perphenazine	Trilafon	8–32	4–64	++	++	+	1:10
piperacetazine	Quide	20–160	5–200	++	++	+	1:10
thioridazine	Mellaril	200–600	20–800	+++	+	++	1:1
trifluoperazine	Stelazine	6–20	2–60	+	+++	+	1:25
triflupromazine	Vesprin	100–150	25–300	++	+++	++	1:3.5
Thioxanthenes							
chlorprothixene	Taractan	50–400	30–600	+++	++	++	1:1
thiothixene	Navane	6–30	6–60	+ to ++	++	++	1:25
Others							
haloperidol	Haldol	6–20	1–100	+	+++	+	1:50
loxapine	Loxitane	60–100	20–250	+	++	+	1:10
molindone	Moban	50–100	15–225	++	+	0	1:10

Note: Adapted from "Drugs and the Treatment of Psychiatric Disorders" by R. J. Baldessarini, in *The Pharmacological Basis of Therapeutics* (7th ed., pp. 403–405) by A. G. Gilman, L. S. Goodman, T. W. Rall, and F. Murad (Eds.), 1985, New York: Macmillan. Copyright 1985 by Macmillan Publishing Co.
*Extreme dosage ranges are occasionally exceeded cautiously and only when appropriate measures have failed.
†Based on data reported by J. M. Davis (1976).

Table 4.3. Neuroleptic Drug Dosages for Children Under
12 Years of Age[a]

Generic Name	Trade Name	Oral Dose (mg/day)
chlorpromazine	Thorazine	10–200
fluphenazine[b]	Prolixin	0.25–16
haloperidol	Haldol	0.25–16
molindone[b]	Moban	1–40
pimozide[c]	Orap	1–7
thioridazine	Mellaril	10–200
thiothixene[b]	Navane	1–40
trifluoperazine[d]	Stelazine	1–20

[a]The most current issue of the *Physicians' Desk Reference* should be consulted for dosage information.
[b]As of 1990, not approved by the Food and Drug Administration in the United States for use with children under 12 years of age.
[c]Not recommended for use in the pediatric age range for any disorder other than Tourette syndrome.
[d]Recommended for use only with children (6–12 years of age) who are hospitalized or under close supervision.

a low-potency agent (e.g., chlorpromazine) to a high-potency neuroleptic (e.g., haloperidol), the dose of the high-potency drug is actually higher in chlorpromazine equivalents than what was being administered initially.

The elimination half-lives of neuroleptic drugs are relatively long (20 to 40 hours), and the biological effects of a single dose are typically present for at least 24 hours. For this reason, neuroleptics are sometimes administered in one oral dose at bedtime after the treatment regimen has stabilized. Once-a-day dosing is not only convenient for the patient (and caregivers), but side effects are sometimes less troublesome with this schedule. Long-lasting dosage forms are also available. These include oral sustained-release chlorpromazine (Thorazine SR) and injectable esterized formulations of fluphenazine (enanthate and decanoate), which have half-lives of 2 to 3 days and 7 to 10 days, respectively. Fluphenazine decanoate injections are generally administered every 2 to 3 weeks. There is also a long-lasting formulation of haloperidol (decanoate), which is administered at 4-week intervals.

EFFICACY

The neuroleptics possess an extraordinary ability to suppress a wide variety of behaviors. For behaviors that pose a threat to self or others, interfere with the ability to perform routine daily functions, or impede social acceptance, reductions in rate, frequency, or severity are likely to be perceived as being therapeutically beneficial. However, when neuroleptic drug therapy results in a concurrent suppression of adaptive behaviors (e.g., verbal expression, social interaction, work or school performance, problem-solving), patient and caregivers may question whether or not the benefits of symptom alleviation are worth the price of impairment of previously normal functions. The clinical picture is complicated by the fact that neuroleptics can also induce a broad spectrum of somatic disorders that range in severity from unpleasant to personally devastating.

We present here in alphabetical order an overview of several of the many psychiatric disorders and target behaviors for which neuroleptic drugs are prescribed. The primary diagnostic features of each disorder are briefly described, as are the symptoms that improve with neuroleptic medication, at least for some individuals.

Aggression

Aggressive behavior takes many forms and includes verbal aggression (cursing, threatening, malicious teasing), object aggression (breaking toys, destroying property), symbolic aggression (feigning physical attack, making offensive gestures), and physical aggression (striking, shoving or tripping other people). In residential facilities, aggressive behavior is one of the most common reasons for prescribing neuroleptic medication. Numerous studies have shown that neuroleptic drugs can suppress aggressive behavior in individuals diagnosed as being mentally retarded (reviewed by Gadow & Poling, 1988), hyperactive (e.g., Gittelman-Klein, Klein, Katz, Saraf & Pollack, 1976; Werry & Aman, 1975), autistic (see Campbell, Anderson, Deutsch & Green, 1984c), or conduct-disordered (e.g., Campbell et al., 1984b). The three most commonly prescribed neuroleptic drugs for the control of aggression in child patients are thioridazine, chlorpromazine, and haloperidol.

Anxiety Disorders

Anxiety disorders are typically treated with antianxiety (see chapter 5) or antidepressant (see chapter 7) medication, depending upon the disorder, but the neuroleptics are also occasionally used for patients whose symptoms are particularly debilitating or are unresponsive to more conventional therapies. Patients undergoing neuroleptic treatment must be apprised of the associated risks, particularly for long-term use.

Autism

Autism is a rare disorder affecting 2 to 4 children in every 10,000. The key features are a lack of responsiveness to other people, which is called autism, serious speech abnormalities (e.g., echolalia, improper use of pronouns, lack of speech, inability to use abstractions), and bizarre mannerisms (resistance to change in the environment, emotional attachment to strange objects, stereotypies). When these symptoms occur before 30 months of age, the disorder is referred to as infantile autism. Most, but certainly not all, children who are autistic score in the mentally retarded range on standardized intelligence tests, although some youngsters possess extraordinary mental abilities. The disorder is much more common in boys and is typically a life-long disability. Although some autistic children are able to achieve economic self-sufficiency in adulthood, most suffer from the residual effects of the condition (social ineptness), and many are provided for in institutional facilities or community placements (e.g., sheltered workshops). Those with higher intellectual ability and better language skills enjoy a more favorable prognosis.

Owing to the early onset of symptoms, pharmacotherapy may be initiated during early childhood. In fact, most of the well-controlled neuroleptic drug studies pertain to preschool-aged autistic children; the findings show that neuroleptic drugs can reduce social withdrawal, hyperactivity, stereotypies, fidgetiness, and abnormal object relations in some patients. Haloperidol is superior to the phenothiazines because it is less likely to cause sedation at optimal doses. Haloperidol has also been shown to increase the effectiveness of a language-based behavior therapy program (Campbell et al., 1978) and appears to facilitate discrimination learning (Anderson et al., 1984). The optimal dose for most preschoolers ranges from 0.5 to 1.0 mg per day. Hypoactive autistic children are not helped by treatment with haloperidol, and their symptoms may even become worse. The duration of treatment is characteristically determined by the degree to which the drug continues to produce a clinically meaningful therapeutic response, which can be assessed only with systematic dosage reductions and drug-free periods.

Hyperactivity (Attention-deficit Hyperactivity Disorder)

Although stimulant drugs are characteristically used to treat hyperactivity (see chapter 6), neuroleptics are sometimes prescribed for this disorder when symptoms are severe. For example, research on intellectually normal hyperactive children (e.g., Gittelman-Klein et al., 1976) has found that thioridazine leads to behavioral improvement, particularly in the area of conduct problems.

Mania

As discussed in chapter 7, lithium is the primary antimanic agent, but the neuroleptics are also helpful. Because the latter have a more rapid calming effect, they are often given in combination with lithium in the initial phase of the illness (see also Drug Interactions).

Organic Mental Syndromes/Disorders

The term *organic mental syndromes/disorders* refers to a variety of conditions whose common feature is a transient or permanent disturbance of mental or behavioral function due to some organic factor (e.g., disease process, substance abuse). A distinction is made between conditions of known (disorder) and unknown (syndrome) etiology. Two of the most common organic mental syndromes are delirium and dementia. Delirium is characterized by a reduced ability to maintain and shift attention, disorganized thinking (manifested by rambling, irrelevant, or incoherent speech), reduced level of consciousness, perceptual disturbances (misinterpretations, illusions, hallucinations), sleep problems, change in normal pattern of psychomotor activity, disorientation to time, place, or person, and memory impairment. The clinical features of dementia are personality changes and impairment of short- and long-term memory, abstract thinking, judgment, and higher cortical function. Both delirium and dementia are fairly common in the elderly. This explains, in part, the extremely high rate of neuroleptic drug prescribing in residential programs for the aged (e.g., Avorn, Dreyer, Connelly & Soumerai, 1989). When treating these disorders, low doses of high-potency neuroleptics are recommended because they are least likely to induce additional mental dulling.

Schizophrenia

Schizophrenia is characterized by unusual and alien sensory perceptions (*hallucinations*, e.g., hearing voices that are not real), misinterpretation of the environment (*delusions*, e.g., the belief that people are following or conspiring against them), or jumbled and disjointed thinking (*thought disorder*, e.g., rambling or pointless speech, failure to keep a train of thought). Individuals with such symptoms often experience many other behavioral changes (sleep problems, overactivity, underactivity, social withdrawal, or very inappropriate social behavior). Schizophrenia is a life-long disorder with variable severity and degree of social, behavioral, and intellectual deterioration. *Florid* (active, easily observed) psychotic symptoms (e.g., hallucinations, delusions) occur in some stage of the illness and are not related to mood disturbance or gross abnormality of brain functioning (e.g., head injury, drug or alcohol abuse). In addition to the florid symptoms, there is chronic evidence of personality change, usually expressed as abnormal affect (e.g., emotional reactions are less intense, limited in scope, or inappropriate to the context of the situation such as laughing about very sad events). Other characteristics are social withdrawal, lack of purpose, and failure to reach potential socially or vocationally. One type of schizophrenia, *catatonia*, is characterized by a mute, withdrawn state in which abnormal postures may be maintained for many hours or by an extreme, excitable, uncontrolled, overactive state. When motor problems have improved, the more classical schizophrenic thought abnormalities usually become more detectable.

The efficacy of neuroleptics for the treatment of acute schizophrenia has been established in scores of studies (reviewed by Klein et al., 1980), some of which have involved hundreds of patients (e.g., National Institutes of Mental Health, 1964). Studies examining the relative efficacy of various treatment approaches for acute schizophrenia have found drug therapy to be only slightly less effective than a combination of drug therapy and psychotherapy, both of which were more effective than psychotherapy alone (May, 1968; Quality Assurance Project, 1984). Electroconvulsive therapy was found to be more effective than psychotherapy but less effective than drug therapy.

No single neuroleptic can be considered the "right" medication for most patients. Some do better with one agent than with another, but the only way to determine this is through trial and error. One of the most important considerations in selecting a drug for a particular patient is the relative risk of specific side effects. For example, if drug-induced hypotension (see Table 4.2) is a clinical concern because the patient has a history of cardiovascular disease, then a low dose–high potency agent (e.g., haloperidol) would be more appropriate than a high dose–low potency neuroleptic (e.g., chlorpromazine). Some acutely psychotic patients may show signs of clinical improvement within 48 hours, but hospitalized schizophrenics may require 3 weeks of neuroleptic treatment before therapeutic effects are evidenced. The full extent of drug response may be manifest only after several weeks to several months of treatment. Some patients are benefitted little by neuroleptic medication or helped only during periodic episodes of symptom exacerbation. Others actually become worse on medication.

At the onset of an acute psychotic episode, the clinician typically attempts to bring the behavioral disturbance under control as soon as possible. When oral preparations are used, the dose is increased rapidly over a few days. Intramuscular injections of neuroleptics can also be used to achieve more immediate results, but one must be attentive to potential adverse reactions (e.g., hypotension, acute dystonic reactions). There is a belief that a rapid increase in dose (e.g., during the first 24 hours of treatment) to unusually high levels, typically with a high-potency agent (a procedure sometimes referred to as *rapid neuroleptization*), leads to more favorable clinical response and a briefer illness. Baldessarini, Cohen & Teicher (1988) note, however, that there is absolutely no empirical support for this practice. After the patient's symptoms have stabilized, dosage can be adjusted to the optimal level, and later, single daily dose administrations can be considered. If patient compliance is a problem, long-acting neuroleptic drug preparations can be used, such as fluphenazine decanoate. General neuroleptic dosage guidelines for adult schizophrenics are presented in the "usual daily oral dose" column in Table 4.2.

Collectively, studies on the dose-response effects of neuroleptics on the acute phase of schizophrenia show a curvilinear relationship (Baldessarini et al., 1988). In chlorpromazine equivalents, both low (<250 mg) and high (>800 mg) daily doses are generally ineffective, whereas moderate doses (300 to 600 mg) appear to produce optimal therapeutic response. Higher doses are thought to be less effective than moderate doses because they are often associated with extrapyramidal reactions (see Untoward Effects), which are interpreted as symptom exacerbation.

Neuroleptic polypharmacy is ill-advised for schizophrenic patients. However, combinations of a neuroleptic and tricyclic antidepressant or lithium are often prescribed for patients with concomitant mood disturbances. A controlled study of tricyclic antidepressants given in combination with neuroleptic medication to "depressed" schizophrenics showed that the antidepressants were not helpful for the treatment of depressive symptoms (Kramer et al., 1989).

Many chronic schizophrenic patients require long-term "maintenance" drug therapy to prevent or postpone the recurrence of periodic episodes of more active symptoms (Davis, 1975; Hogarty & Ulrich, 1977). Often dosage can be reduced for short periods of time (weeks to months) between acute episodes without signs of relapse. Maintenance treatment can be made less inconvenient and more effective (by eliminating noncompliance) by using monthly injections of fluphenazine decanoate or haloperidol decanoate (Beresford & Ward, 1987; Johnson, 1984; Kane, 1983). Even low doses can be very effective (Marder, Hawes & Van

Patten, 1986). Unfortunately, although depot injections are more clinically advantageous than oral preparations, the 2-year relapse rate is still approximately 30% (Johnson, 1976; Watt, 1975).

Children and Adolescents. Childhood schizophrenia is a rare disorder and a separate diagnostic entity from infantile autism. One important difference between the two disorders is that autistic children do not experience auditory or visual hallucinations or delusions, whereas most schizophrenic children do have these symptoms (Green et al., 1984). Whether neuroleptics suppress hallucinations, delusions, and disordered thought in schizophrenic prepubertal children is not well documented, and cases of drug failure are not uncommon. Neuroleptics that are more "stimulating" (e.g., thiothixene, haloperidol) are generally preferred.

There are a few methodologically sound studies of the efficacy of neuroleptic medication for the treatment of schizophrenia during adolescence. One of the better studies, conducted by Pool, Bloom, Mielke, Roniger and Gallant (1976), showed that haloperidol and loxapine were superior to placebo in controlling psychotic symptoms. Similarly, Realmuto, Erickson, Yellin, Hopwood and Greenberg (1984) studied adolescents receiving thioridazine and thiothixene and found that (compared with baseline) treatment with either medication was associated with a decrease in anxiety, tension, excitement, and hallucinations, and, to a modest extent, cognitive disorganization. The optimal doses of thioridazine and thiothixene were 3.3 mg/kg per day and 0.30 mg/kg per day, respectively. Unfortunately, despite diminution of these symptoms, the youths "continued to be quite impaired" (p. 441), and by the end of the study only one-half were considered to be improved.

Self-Injurious Behavior

The term *self-injurious behavior* (SIB) is generally applied to a repetitive pattern of behavior (e.g., banging, biting, scratching, gouging) that results in tissue damage to one's own body. Self-injurious behavior is most commonly observed in individuals who are severely or profoundly mentally retarded or autistic, but it is also associated with some degenerative and central nervous system disorders and severe forms of other psychiatric disorders such as schizophrenia and obsessive compulsive disorder. Studies of mentally retarded people in institutions (e.g., Griffin, Williams, Stark, Altmeyer & Mason, 1986; Schroeder, Schroeder, Smith & Dalldorf, 1978) indicate that approximately 10% to 15% exhibit self-injurious behavior. Despite the seriousness of this disorder and our heartfelt reactions to it, there are few well-conducted studies that have examined the effectiveness of neuroleptics, even though these drugs are generally considered to be therapeutic (reviewed by Farber, 1987; Singh & Millichamp, 1985).

Several phenothiazines and haloperidol have been shown to suppress self-injurious behavior; however, because it has multiple etiologies, both psychological (Durand, 1987) and biological (Schroeder, Bicker & Richmond, 1986), careful consideration should be given to the possibility that specific environmental events are maintaining this behavior when formulating a treatment plan. A variety of behavioral techniques are effective (reviewed by Romanczyk, 1986), and Durand (1982) showed that haloperidol in combination with mild punishment was more effective than either treatment used alone in reducing self-injurious behavior in a profoundly mentally retarded adolescent.

Stereotypies

Stereotypies (e.g., body rocking, arm flapping, undirected vocalization) are generally defined as intentional, repetitive behaviors that serve no constructive or socially acceptable purpose. They differ from motor and vocal tics, which are considered to be involuntary but can nevertheless be suppressed for varying lengths of time. Stereotypies are fairly common in severely to profoundly mentally retarded or autistic individuals. Self-injurious behavior is considered to be a type of stereotypy by some authorities.

Stereotypies are of concern to caregivers because they interfere with educational and habilitative efforts and can be an impediment to normalization, in that bizarre behaviors are generally perceived in a negative way by others. There is now substantial evidence that thioridazine reduces levels of stereotypic behavior in mentally retarded people (reviewed by Aman & Singh, 1983). Whether drug-induced reductions in stereotypic behaviors lead to performance gains in other areas is unknown. It is noteworthy that Singh and Aman (1981) found that a low dose (2.5 mg/kg) of thioridazine was as effective as higher therapeutic doses in controlling stereotypies. Interestingly, although Zimmermann and Heistad (1982) found that withdrawal from thioridazine led to a marked increase in stereotypic behavior in mentally retarded adults housed in a large state institution, stereotypies were rarely the primary reason for prescribing medication in the first place.

Stuttering

There are several published reports on the effect of haloperidol on stuttering (e.g., Burns, Brady & Kuruvilla, 1978; Quinn & Peachey, 1973; Tapia, 1969; Wells & Malcolm, 1971). In general, the findings from these studies and case reports indicate that haloperidol can suppress or diminish stuttering in some individuals. Why haloperidol should have this effect on stutterers is unclear, and, as for all disorders for which this drug is prescribed, careful consideration must be given to the associated risks of treatment versus the benefits. Interestingly, in an uncontrolled study Fisher, Kerbeshian and Burd (1986) found that haloperidol also had a marked effect on facilitating language development in nonautistic children with pervasive developmental disorder.

Tourette Syndrome

Tourette syndrome can be an extremely debilitating condition and is characterized by multiple, frequently changing motor and vocal (phonic) tics. The diagnosis is based on the following criteria: (a) onset before age 21 years; (b) multiple motor and one or more vocal tics, although not necessarily concurrent; (c) tics occur many times a day, nearly every day or intermittently through a period of more than 1 year; and (d) waxing and waning of symptoms (i.e., variations in intensity and type of tics over time). Motor tics can be separated into two groups: *simple* (fast, darting, and meaningless muscle spasms) and *complex* (slower and more purposeful). Examples of simple motor tics are eye blinking, nose twitching, grimacing, shoulder shrugging, arm or head jerking, finger movements, jaw snapping, and rapid jerking of any body part. Complex motor tics include such things as clapping, throwing, hopping, self-mutilation, touching objects, bending to touch the floor, sticking out the tongue, *echopraxia* (imitating what one has just seen), and so forth. Vocal tics are also varied and include *simple* tics (e.g., whistling, sniffling, barking, grunting, coughing, and so forth), *complex vocal tics* (e.g., saying words, phrases, or statements), *coprolalia* (saying obscene or aggressive words or statements), *palilalia* (repeating one's own words), and *echolalia* (repeating the words of others). Tics range from mild to severe and show extreme variability in type, frequency, and severity over time. They are frequently situation specific (e.g., may be controlled in school but occur at a distressing level at home, particularly right after school). In addition to motor and vocal tics, approximately one-half of all diagnosed cases of Tourette syndrome also experience the behavioral symptoms of hyperactivity. Learning disabilities and academic underachievement are common, as are obsessions and compulsions.

Since the 1960s the drug of first choice for the treatment of Tourette syndrome has been haloperidol (reviewed by Shapiro, Shapiro, Young & Feinberg, 1988). Approximately 80% of all patients show some initial benefit from this medication but, primarily because of side effects, far fewer (approximately 20% to 30%) take the drug for extended periods of time. Haloperidol is very effective at low doses. Patients are generally started on a dose of 0.25 to 0.5 mg/day (administered at bedtime), which is increased every 4 or 5 days (at no more than 0.5 mg increments) to an average daily dose of 3 to 4 mg (range = 2 to 10 mg). At low doses, many patients experience a complete remission of symptoms and few adverse reactions.

The withdrawal of haloperidol may lead to an exacerbation of symptoms to a level far worse than before the onset of medication, which may last for up to 2 to 3 months. Conversely, some patients may show improvement following drug discontinuation only to worsen later and gradually improve again. The withdrawal of medication may also be greeted with some relief because side effects such as cognitive blunting dissipate. For these reasons, evaluating the need to continue treatment is a complex process. Not only should the patient be prepared for these possibilities, but also drug-free periods or dosage reductions should be scheduled to assess the need to continue medication.

Fluphenazine is an effective substitute for haloperidol (Singer, Gammon & Quaskey, 1986). It is also less likely to cause troublesome side effects at therapeutic doses (2 to 15 mg/day).

Pimozide (Orap) is a powerful neuroleptic shown to be effective for the treatment of Tourette syndrome, and controlled studies suggest that it is only slightly less effective than haloperidol and is less sedating (Shapiro et al., 1989). Treatment is typically initiated with a dose of 1 mg per day, which is gradually increased (1 mg per week) to an average dose of 7 mg per day (range: 2 to 12 mg). Pimozide can have an adverse effect on heart function, and therefore an EKG should be obtained prior to treatment.

The behavioral concomitants of Tourette syndrome (e.g., hyperactivity, obsessions, compulsions) and its psychological sequelae (e.g., embarrassment, social rejection, anxiety from not being in control of one's own body) and associated academic impediments (both drug-induced and preexisting) necessitate complex and broad-spectrum interventions, to which neuroleptic medication can be a valuable adjunct. The clinician must ensure that the patient's emotional needs are being attended to (Bauer & Shea, 1984) and that appropriate treatment is directed toward each target symptom.

UNTOWARD EFFECTS

In addition to their ability to alter mood, thought processes, and behavior, neuroleptics affect a number of bodily functions by their ability to interfere with the actions of at least several important neurotransmitters (reviewed by Baldessarini, 1985b; Klein, Gittleman-Klein, Quit-kin & Rifkin, 1980). People generally develop a tolerance for many of the adverse reactions associated with neuroleptic medication; death is a highly unlikely consequence of overdosage (as in suicide attempts), and serious toxic effects are rare. Neuroleptics can nevertheless impair adaptive behavior and produce a sometimes irreversible neurological disorder (tardive dyskinesia).

Sedation (e.g., drowsiness, lethargy) is a very common side effect of the low-potency neuroleptics (e.g., thioridazine, chlorpromazine) but is much less troublesome with high-potency agents (see Table 4.2). Tolerance to sedative effects typically develops within days to a few weeks after the onset of treatment.

Neuroleptic drugs produce a variety of autonomic nervous system reactions that include blurred vision, dry mouth, nausea, decreased sweating and salivation, nasal stuffiness, dizziness, constipation and inhibition of ejaculation (but not necessarily erection). The latter problem is more commonly associated with thioridazine (reviewed by Se-graves, 1989). Neuroleptics can impair various aspects of sexual function in both males and females (reviewed by Shen, Sata & Hofstatter, 1984). Autonomic nervous system reactions (i.e., anticholinergic effects) are more likely to be caused by the less potent phenothiazines (e.g., thioridazine, chlorpromazine).

Another relatively frequent side effect is *orthostatic hypotension* (lowered blood pressure upon standing erect). Persons experiencing such a reaction may feel faint, dizzy, or weak, especially when they get up in the morning and may actually fall. This effect usually appears during the first week of treatment but is seldom a serious problem because tolerance develops rather quickly. Nevertheless, a mild form of this reaction may continue as long as the patient is taking medication. Orthostatic hypotension is more likely to occur with thioridazine and chlorpromazine than with haloperidol (see Table 4.2).

The endocrine system can also be affected by treatment with the phenothiazines. For example, increased prolactin secretion may occur while on medication. Tolerance to this reaction does not develop, but it is reversible upon drug discontinuation. Drug-induced changes in the release of growth hormones may account for frequent reports of increased appetite and weight gain associated with treatment with phenothiazines.

Jaundice is observed in less than 1% of the patients treated with chlorpromazine and is generally considered a hypersensitivity reaction (Klein et al., 1980). It is typically mild and commonly occurs between the second and fourth week of treatment. If jaundice occurs, medication is usually (but not always) terminated and another drug is substituted.

Skin reactions are fairly common, with urticaria or dermatitis re-ported in about 5% of patients receiving phenothiazines. This effect usually occurs within the first to fifth week of treatment, clearing up when medication is discontinued. Most skin rashes are self-limiting. *Phototoxicity* (also called *photosensitivity* by some clinicians) is another type of skin reaction. For some patients taking phenothiazines, expo-sure to the sun for even a few minutes results in a severe sunburn. Such damage can be prevented by simply keeping clothed areas well covered and using a sunscreen on skin exposed to sunlight.

Long-term exposure to phenothiazines, particularly at higher doses, can result in abnormal concentrations of *melanin* (skin pigmentation). This reaction (which is rare and most commonly associated with chlor-promazine) is characterized by gray-blue patches of skin in areas ex-posed to the sun. Opacities in the cornea and in the lens of the eye are present in some patients treated with neuroleptic medication. Gowdey, Coleman, and Crawford (1985) conducted a study of opacities in men-tally retarded adults treated with phenothiazines and found that opac-ities were (a) more common in patients with brown eyes; (b) not likely to impair vision; (c) more related to monthly drug intake than total drug exposure; and (d) less common in patients receiving concurrent antiepileptic drugs (phenobarbital, phenytoin, primidone), presumably because of the latter drugs' liver-enzyme-inducing properties (which may lead to lower phenothiazine blood levels). Skin pigments can also concentrate in the retina of the eye *(pigmentary retinopathy)*, an effect reported primarily in cases of thioridazine treatment with doses in ex-cess of 1,000 mg/day.

Neuroleptics, particularly when administered in high or rapidly in-creasing dosages, can cause tonic-clonic (grand mal) seizures. This problem can be easily managed by making a slight decrease in dosage. Low-to-moderate dosages of neuroleptics are unlikely to precipitate sei-zures in patients with seizure disorders if they are receiving an ade-quate amount of antiepileptic medication or in seizure-free patients with a history of epilepsy (James, 1986).

Neuroleptics can also alter body temperature, producing either a mild increase or a decrease *(hypothermia)*. In the latter case, patients may complain of "feeling cold."

Extrapyramidal Syndromes

Perhaps the most disquieting and alarming side effects of neurolep-tics are the extrapyramidal syndromes, disorders that involve certain motor areas of the brain called the *extrapyramidal tract*. The various nu-clei and nerve fibers that make up this structure control and coordinate motor activities, especially walking, posture, muscle tone, and patterns of movement. Drugs that affect the extrapyramidal tract can cause spasms in skeletal muscles and changes in body posture, facial expression, and movement of the limbs. Four different extrapyramidal syndromes are associated with the use of major tranquilizers: parkinsonian syndrome, akathisia, acute dystonic reactions, and tardive dyskinesia. These side effects are most commonly associated with haloperidol, trifluoperazine, or fluphenazine and are less likely to occur with thioridazine (see Table 4.2).

Parkinsonian Syndrome. The parkinsonian syndrome (parkinsonism) caused by the neuroleptics mimics the symptoms of Parkinson disease. The syndrome is characterized by *bradykinesia* (extreme slowness of movement) and *akinesia* (absence or loss of the power of voluntary movement). The latter is associated with muscular weakness, aches, and general tiredness and, in more severe forms, depression, loss of motivation, and an inability to perform repetitive movements such as walking or working. The patient may appear depressed, with a mask-like facial expression that caregivers may refer to as "looking like a zombie." Other symptoms include muscle rigidity, stooped posture, tremor, drooling, a shuffling walk without free swing of the arms, and "pill rolling." The latter refers to movements of the hand as if the patient is rolling a pill between his or her fingers. An early sign for the onset of the parkinsonian syndrome is small, crabbed handwriting. In a large sample of psychiatric patients treated with phenothiazines, Ayd (1961) reported the prevalence of the parkinsonian syndrome to be 15%. It is more common in women and in elderly patients (where it may be mistaken for depression or dementia).

With regard to clinical management, some patients respond to dosage reduction, whereas others require antiparkinsonian agents such as amantadine (Symmetrel), bromocriptine (Parlodel), trihexyphenidyl (Artane), and benztropine (Cogentin). Some antiparkinsonian drugs (e.g., trihexyphenidyl, benztropine) have significant anticholinergic activity and can impair memory and the ability to learn new material. These adverse effects on mental ability have important implications for the treatment of elderly patients (McEvoy et al., 1987). The period of maximal risk for the onset of parkinsonism is during the first month of medication.

There is a rare disorder that resembles a severe case of parkinsonism called *neuroleptic malignant syndrome.* Its primary features are fever, severe extrapyramidal symptoms (e.g., rigidity, dyskinesias), and autonomic dysregulation (e.g., excessive heart rate, unstable blood pressure, profuse sweating, difficulty breathing) or two of these symptoms in combination with one of the following: altered consciousness (e.g., delirium, mutism, stupor, coma), an abnormally large number of white blood cells, or high serum levels of creatine kinase (Pope, Keck & McElroy, 1986). Rosebush and Stewart (1989) described their patients who experienced neuroleptic malignant syndrome as having a frightened facial expression owing to their inability to speak and a sense of impending doom, which produced overwhelming anxiety. Neuroleptic malignant syndrome can occur within hours or months after the onset of drug therapy, is associated primarily with high-potency neuroleptics such as haloperidol, thiothixene, and long-acting fluphenazine derivatives, and is fatal in approximately 10% of the cases (Shalev, Hermesh & Munitz, 1989). Neuroleptic malignant syndrome was once considered to be rare, but it is now believed to occur in 1% to 2% of hospitalized psychiatric patients treated with neuroleptics (Pope et al., 1986). Medication should be stopped immediately when the signs of this disorder first appear. The reaction may last from 5 to 10 days after drug withdrawal. The administration of amantadine, dantrolene (Dantrium), or bromocriptine may be helpful (Coons, Hillman & Marshall, 1982; Mueller, Vester & Fermaglich, 1983), but their efficacy has been questioned by others (Rosebush & Stewart, 1989).

Akathisia. This reaction is characterized by involuntary motor restlessness. The patient is unable to sit still, is constantly fidgeting, and appears to be agitated. In a recent discussion of diagnostic problems, Barnes and Braude (1985) note that the most objective observable features of akathisia are rocking from foot to foot (while standing) and walking in place. Akathisia, however, can be manifested solely as a subjective feeling (a compelling need to move) that can be extremely uncomfortable. It occurs in approximately 20% of adult psychotic patients treated with neuroleptics (Ayd, 1961) and may be easily misdiagnosed in patients who are unable to adequately describe an inner feeling of discomfort (e.g., Kumar, 1979). In some patients, it may also be difficult to distinguish akathisia from tardive dyskinesia (see Munetz & Cornes, 1983).

Akathisia responds to dosage reduction, and in cases in which it occurs in conjunction with severe parkinsonism, anticholinergic medication is helpful (Braude, Barnes & Gore, 1983). For most patients, however, treatment with anticholinergics is of little value. There are reports that propranolol (Lipinski, Zubenko, Cohen & Barreira, 1984) and short-term treatment with benzodiazepine antianxiety agents provide relief for some patients. The period of maximal risk for developing akathisia is the first 2 months of drug therapy.

Acute Dystonic Reactions. Acute dystonic reactions are characterized by abrupt muscle spasms of the tongue, face, neck, and back. Some examples are facial grimacing, *oculogyric crisis* (fixed upward gaze), *torti-*

collis (a twisting of the neck muscles), *retrocollis* (head turned to back), and *opisthotonos* (arching of back). The tongue may be protruded or the teeth tightly clenched. In rare cases, the patient may have difficulty swallowing. Although this reaction responds well to treatment, it can be terrifying for both patient and caregivers. Acute dystonic reactions are more common with high-potency neuroleptics such as haloperidol and trifluoperazine than with other neuroleptics. They occur in 5% to 10% of Tourette syndrome patients treated with haloperidol (Shapiro et al., 1988) and in 40% to 50% of psychiatric patients receiving high-potency neuroleptics (Arana, Goff, Baldessarini & Keepers, 1988). Such reactions are more apt to occur in young male patients and are relatively rare in individuals over the age of 45.

A patient having a severe reaction should receive immediate medical attention. Intravenous or intramuscular injections of diphenhydramine (Benadryl) or an anticholinergic agent provide prompt relief of symptoms; if this treatment is followed by oral doses of benztropine or trihexyphenidyl, there is no need to discontinue neuroleptic medication. When anticholinergic drugs are administered at the onset of high-potency neuroleptic treatment, the incidence of adverse dystonic reactions drops appreciably (6% to 10%) (Arana et al., 1988), but this procedure is controversial because it exposes some patients to a drug they may not need. The period of maximal risk for acute dystonic reactions is the first 5 days of neuroleptic treatment (Ayd, 1961).

Tardive Dyskinesia. Tardive dyskinesia typically appears late, often months after drug therapy has been initiated, and may not be evident until medication is discontinued. It is characterized by rhythmic, repetitive stereotypic movements that appear to be involuntary but can usually be inhibited. Some of the more common features are sucking and smacking movements of the lips, side-to-side shifting of the chin (giving the appearance of a cow "chewing its cud"), thrusting the tongue in and out of the mouth ("fly-catching" fashion), sudden flying out of the arms, moving toes up and down, fingers in and out ("piano playing"), and jerking movements of the body. These symptoms range in severity from barely detectable to crippling. In more severe cases they can interfere with eating, swallowing, wearing dentures, walking, and even breathing and can be so unsightly that they become a serious impediment to rehabilitation and social adjustment. Eyelid and tongue tremors appear to be early signs of the disorder (Gardos, Perenyi, Cole, Samu & Kallos, 1983). Tardive dyskinesia is most common among patients who receive large dosages of neuroleptic medication over extended periods of time. Prevalence figures for this adverse reaction range as high as 15% to 30% among psychiatric patients.

There is no one best method for treating tardive dyskinesia. When the disorder appears while the person is on medication, the dose should be gradually reduced and treatment terminated, or, if psychotic symptoms reappear, use the smallest dose necessary for clinical management. The addition of a benzodiazepine (see chapter 5) may allow the neuroleptic dose to be lowered even more. For individuals who develop tardive dyskinesia after treatment has been terminated, a variety of drugs have been touted as helping some patients, but no single agent is currently recognized as being clinically effective for the long-term management of severe tardive dyskinesia (Gardos et al., 1987). Unfortunately, anticholinergic drugs appear only to aggravate the condition (Chouinard, Montigny & Annable, 1979).

Tardive dyskinesia can persist indefinitely after medication is terminated, but at least one-half of the patients experience gradual improvement over time after medication has been stopped. Most experience at least partial remission. When tardive dyskinesia symptoms occur after drug withdrawal and abate spontaneously within 12 to 16 weeks, the disorder is sometimes referred to as *withdrawal* tardive dyskinesia. If symptoms continue for a longer period of time, the condition is said to be *persistent*. Several steps can be taken to minimize the risk of developing tardive dyskinesia: (a) use the minimal effective dose of neuroleptic medication, (b) examine patients frequently for early signs of tardive dyskinesia, and (c) administer anticholinergic drugs only when necessary and for limited periods of time.

In Children

The side effects of neuroleptics in children are similar to those reported in adults. Sedative effects (drowsiness, lethargy, and apathy) are quite common with chlorpromazine, but tolerance usually develops within several days to a few weeks. Dosage reduction may be necessary in some cases. It is noteworthy that irritability and excitability are also possible adverse effects of neuroleptic medication. Diarrhea, upset stomach, dry mouth, blurred vision, constipation, urinary retention, and abdominal pain occur in some patients. A number of studies report increased appetite or weight gain, or both, during drug treatment. Skin reactions are infrequent.

Katz et al. (1975) state that, in their experience with hyperactive children, the side effects of thioridazine were frequent and severe. Drowsiness was the most common adverse reaction that was difficult to manage. If the dose was reduced, the drowsiness was less severe, but the therapeutic response was weaker. Many children developed enuresis and had to be taken off medication. Increased appetite was also common, as were puffiness around the eyes and mild dry mouth. Stomachache, nausea, and vomiting necessitated dosage reduction in a number of children. Other side effects included nosebleed, mild tremor, and orthostatic hypotension. Some children who reacted well to thioridazine later developed changes in temperament. They became irritable, moody, and belligerent, and medication eventually had to be stopped.

Extrapyramidal syndromes are frequently reported in studies using haloperidol to control behavior disorders in children. Clinicians manage these side effects by administering an anticholinergic agent either at the beginning of drug treatment (a practice that is controversial) or after symptoms appear. Although haloperidol is usually not associated with sedative effects, drowsiness has sometimes been reported in studies of children. Other side effects include nausea, ataxia, slurred speech, and weight gain.

Perhaps the most controversial side effect of the neuroleptics is cognitive and academic impairment. This issue is controversial because studies in this area have not been particularly well designed (reviewed by Aman, 1978). Nevertheless, there are good examples of research on the use of neuroleptics for hyperactive (e.g., Sprague, Barnes & Werry, 1970; Werry & Aman, 1975) and mentally retarded (e.g., Wysocki, Fuqua, Davis & Breuning, 1981) individuals, which strongly suggest that mental impairment is a definite possibility. It is important, therefore, to monitor adaptive behavior during dosage adjustment and to assess the extent to which desirable behaviors may be adversely affected.

DRUG INTERACTIONS

Neuroleptics can prolong and intensify the effects of central nervous system depressants such as hypnotics, sedatives, analgesics, antihistamines, narcotics, and alcohol. Many over-the-counter products contain these drugs, including cold remedies. Some neuroleptics, such as thioridazine, have anticholinergic effects, which are additive when given in combination with other drugs that have anticholinergic properties (e.g., tricyclic antidepressants, antiparkinsonian agents). Some drugs such as sedatives (e.g., phenobarbital) and antiepileptics (e.g., phenytoin, carbamazepine) induce liver enzymes that increase the rate of drug metabolism, resulting in lower neuroleptic blood levels. In one study, haloperidol blood levels dropped 60% when carbamazepine (see chapter 8) was added to the treatment regimen (Jann et al., 1985). There are a few reports indicating that lithium may interact synergistically with neuroleptics, particularly haloperidol, resulting in brain damage (Cohen

& Cohen, 1974) or extrapyramidal side effects (Addonizio, 1985). However, many patients are apparently treated effectively with this drug combination (Tupin & Schuller, 1978).

CONCLUDING COMMENT

The neuroleptics are among the most widely prescribed psychotropic medications. They are used to treat a wide range of behavior disorders, and they have been used effectively with millions of patients. Unfortunately, all of these drugs are capable of producing a range of adverse reactions, including behavioral impairment and motor disturbances. Because of this, decisions concerning the use of any neuroleptic must be made on the basis of a careful risk–benefit analysis for individual patients. Prolonged treatment with these agents appears to be justified only when a patient derives significant overall gain from the medication and when no superior alternative treatment is available.

Chapter 5

Sedatives, Hypnotics, and Anxiolytics

Drugs considered in this chapter are primarily prescribed to induce sleep (a *hypnotic* action) or calm the patient (a *sedative* action). The most common primary diagnosis resulting in hypnotic drug therapy is *insomnia*. This condition is one of the major categories of sleep disorders (Association of Professional Sleep Societies, 1987; American Psychiatric Association, 1987). As sedatives or anxiolytics, these drugs are mainly prescribed for *anxiety* (i.e., as *anxiolytics*), a diverse set of conditions whose major component is fear. Many of the drugs considered in this chapter are also used in the treatment of epilepsy (see chapter 8).

Modern medicine's introduction to sedative–hypnotics began with the recognition of potassium bromide's ability to depress the central nervous system (CNS). Use of this compound to treat epilepsy in the 1850s coincided with some of the earliest pharmacological experiments on the most important hypnotic of the nineteenth century, chloral hydrate. This drug, introduced clinically in 1869, was the first safe hypnotic and soon became widely accepted. Although initial understanding of its mechanism of action proved incorrect (early pharmacologists believed it released chloroform in the blood), its effectiveness prompted testing of related synthetic compounds. Chloral hydrate enjoyed prominence for 30 years in spite of its foul taste and its tendency to produce gastrointestinal upset. Chloral hydrate was followed by the introduction of other successful hypnotics such as paraldehyde, urethan, and sulfanol, all before 1900.

Barbital, the first of the barbiturates to be used clinically, was introduced by F. Bayer and Company in 1903. The drug class name, barbiturate, has been variously attributed to the day barbituric acid was synthesized (St. Barbara's Day) or the name of the woman who was the object of the discoverer's affection (Sneader, 1985). Once the superiority of barbital was recognized, thousands of other barbiturates were synthesized and tested. The barbiturates lacked some of the more aversive side effects of the chloral derivatives and soon replaced all other hypnotics except chloral hydrate. One of the most successful barbiturates, phenobarbital, was synthesized in 1911 and proved to be both a popular sedative–hypnotic and a valuable antiepileptic agent (see chapter 8). Phenobarbital was followed by amylobarbital (Amytal), quinalbarbital/secobarbital (Seconal), and pentobarbital (Nembutal) in the 1920s. Prior to the introduction of the neuroleptics in the 1950s, high doses of barbiturates were often prescribed for psychotic patients to induce sedation. Barbiturates monopolized the sedative–hypnotic marketplace until the introduction of the benzodiazepines in 1961.

The first benzodiazepine to be discovered was chlordiazepoxide (Librium). It was patented in 1958 and underwent extensive clinical trials over the next 3 years. Initial reports suggested that the drug had superior antianxiety properties and produced few significant side effects (Sneader, 1985). Chlordiazepoxide soon became quite popular, and several related benzodiazepines, including diazepam (Valium), were developed and marketed. Used to treat a variety of complaints ranging from mild stress to severe anxiety, the benzodiazepines became in terms of sales volume the most successful pharmaceuticals of all time. Although in recent years their high abuse potential and the persistence of their hypnotic effect have alarmed many physicians, the benzodiazepines still account for a substantial proportion of all prescriptions written each year in the United States.

SEDATIVE–HYPNOTIC PHARMACOLOGY

Sedative-hypnotic drugs may be pharmacologically grouped into benzodiazepines, barbiturates, chloral derivatives, and several unrelated prescription and over-the-counter medications (Sepinwall & Cook, 1978). The benzodiazepines are by far the most popular sedative–hypnotics used today. In addition to their sedative and hypnotic effects, they are prescribed for movement disorders and as muscle relaxants, preanesthetics, and antiepileptics. The degree to which the anxiolytic, sedative, and hypnotic effects represent different processes and mechanisms of action is unresolved. Because the different benzodiazepines share many characteristics, their pharmacological effects and properties will be considered together.

Benzodiazepines

Benzodiazepines are usually given orally and have a rapid onset of action. They are readily absorbed from the stomach, although some do not enter the bloodstream in their original form. There is also rapid uptake into the central nervous system and somewhat slower distribution into fat and muscle. Peak blood concentrations for individual drugs are achieved from 0.5 to 8 hours after oral ingestion. The duration of action for benzodiazepines spans a broad range, with half-lives from 2 to 200 hours for the drugs and their active metabolites. Metabolism is primarily via microsomal enzyme systems in the liver (Harvey, 1985). Because several benzodiazepines undergo biotransformation into active metabolites with radically different half-lives, the half-life of the parent compound is often not well correlated with the duration of action of the drug.

Dose and Schedule of Administration. Benzodiazepines are subject to the Federal Controlled Substances Act as Schedule IV drugs. They are limited to distribution by prescription only. There are numerous benzodiazepines, with widely differing potencies. The specific benzodiazepine drugs are listed in Table 5.1 along with their approximate dose ranges. In general, benzodiazepines are produced in tablet, oral solution, and/ or capsule form. A few, including diazepam, lorazepam, and midazolam, are available for acute administration by injection.

Benzodiazepines are commonly given three or four times per day in divided doses (see Table 5.1). Initial doses are usually low, with gradual increases across several days, until the therapeutically effective dose is reached. With continuous use, blood levels may increase across time, allowing fewer daily doses or reduction of total amount. In prescribing benzodiazepines it is important to ascertain whether the patient has a history of drug abuse, to use the minimal effective dose, and to establish an a priori limit on duration of treatment (Dimijian, 1984).

Mechanism of Action. Most recent evidence suggests that the mechanism of action for the therapeutic effects of benzodiazepines lies in the enhancement of inhibition produced by the neurotransmitter gamma-aminobutyric acid (GABA). In short, these drugs are thought to act to increase the effect of a major neurotransmitter whose role is to suppress central nervous system activity. Potentiation of GABA's inhibitory function, rather than direct action on excitatory systems, may account for the benzodiazepine's wide margin of safety (Harvey, 1985). Specific sites of action (receptors) for benzodiazepines as well as competitive antagonists for these receptors have been discovered in the cerebral cortex, midbrain, and limbic system (Skolnick & Paul, 1982).

Table 5.1. Benzodiazepines

Benzodiazepine	Trade Name	Primary Therapeutic Application	Daily Oral Adult Dose Range (mg/day)
alprazolam	Xanax	Anxiolytic (panic)	0.75–8
chlordiazepoxide	Librium	Anxiolytic	10–100
chlorazepate	Tranxene	Anxiolytic	3.75–30
clonazepam	Klonopin	Antiepileptic (panic)	1.5–20
diazepam	Valium	Anxiolytic	5–40
flunitrazepam	Rohypnol[a]	Hypnotic	1–4
flurazepam	Dalmane	Hypnotic	15–30
halazepam	Paxipam	Anxiolytic	60–160
lorazepam	Ativan	Anxiolytic (panic)	2–4
midazolam	Versed	Anxiolytic	2–5
nitrazepam	Mogadon[a]	Hypnotic	5–10
oxazepam	Serax	Anxiolytic	30–120
prazepam	Centrax	Anxiolytic	20–60
temazepam	Restoril	Hypnotic	15–30
triazolam	Halcion	Hypnotic	0.125–0.5

[a] Europe only

High concentrations of receptors in specific brain locations may be related to their pharmacological effect: anxiolytic effects in the amygdala, hippocampus, and olfactory bulb and sedative effects in the reticular formation, pons, and medulla (Connor, 1984).

The therapeutic efficacy of benzodiazepines is primarily due to effects on the central nervous system, where they decrease general activity without being neuronal depressants. Arousal is decreased after benzodiazepine administration, as is the magnitude of response to external stimulation. Electroencephalograph (EEG) recordings show an increase in slower frequencies, as would be expected with an effective hypnotic. According to EEG records, there appears to be a dose-dependent progression from sedation to hypnosis to stupor. Muscle relaxation and ataxia occur at moderate doses of most benzodiazepines, although there is tolerance to these effects (Harvey, 1985).

Untoward Effects. The most common complaint during benzodiazepine therapy is drowsiness. This may or may not be an unwanted effect, but one advantage of benzodiazepines over other sedative–hypnotics is their ability to produce therapeutic effects at doses that do not cause general depression of activity. Other side effects include ataxia, fatigue, syncope (i.e., brief loss of consciousness caused by inadequate blood to the brain), slurred speech, tremor, vertigo, constipation, hypotension, rash, nausea, headache, and altered libido. These effects are usually mild and often disappear after the first few days of treatment. Motor performance is adversely affected at the time of peak plasma level and subsequently driving ability may be severely impaired. *Anterograde amnesia*, that is, loss of memory of recent events, is occasionally reported. This particular effect may in fact be a therapeutic goal rather than an unwanted side effect, as when benzodiazepines are used as a preanesthetic. Rebound phenomena, such as insomnia, anxiety, excitement, and muscle spasticity, may occur after withdrawal of the drug. Should these phenomena occur during drug treatment (a *paradoxical reaction*), drug treatment should be discontinued. The incidence of allergic reactions is low with benzodiazepines (Harvey, 1985).

Physical Dependence. Of great concern are the adverse effects associated with physical dependence produced by long-term benzodiazepine use. Although the abuse liability appears to be lower for benzodiazepines than for other sedative–hypnotics (e.g., meprobamate and barbiturates), the withdrawal syndromes are similar. Typical abstinence signs include tachycardia, tremor, vomiting, sweating, cramps, and seizures. Gradual dosage reduction may decrease the severity of these symptoms.

Drug Interactions. Benzodiazepines have a wide margin of safety and are rarely fatal even when consumed in large quantities (e.g., in accidental overdose or suicide attempts). Unfortunately, toxicity increases when benzodiazepines are combined with other drugs. When adverse drug interactions occur, they usually (but not exclusively) involve chlordiazepoxide or diazepam. Alcohol is the most common drug showing adverse effects in combination with benzodiazepines. Lethal dose levels of benzodiazepine–alcohol combinations are substantially lower than for either drug alone. In addition, coma, respiratory depression, and cardiovascular damage increase dramatically in likelihood and severity when other central nervous system depressants are taken concomitantly. Cigarette smoking may decrease the sedative effects of benzodiazepines (McEvoy, 1988).

Some drugs decrease the rate of metabolism and elimination of benzodiazepines and thus increase their effects. For example, disulfiram, cimetidine, and erythromycin are known to potentiate the action of benzodiazepines; thus patients should be carefully monitored when these drugs are used in combination with any benzodiazepine. Benzodiazepine absorption may be decreased by antacids (McEvoy, 1988). There is some evidence that amitryptiline increases levels of benzodiazepine in blood.

Benzodiazepines also may change the potency or duration of action of other drugs. Levodopa and phenytoin (Dilantin) may be less effective with concomitant benzodiazepine use. Because digoxin blood levels (and effects) sometimes increase following diazepam treatment, they should be monitored closely, especially in the elderly. Combinations of benzodiazepines and diphenhydramine in pregnant women should be avoided (McEvoy, 1988).

Barbiturates

The barbiturates have lost the prominence they once enjoyed as therapeutic agents for the treatment of anxiety and insomnia and as preanesthetics. They are still employed for a few specialized uses, including the treatment of epilepsy (see chapter 8).

Because most barbiturates are taken orally, absorption is dependent upon gastrointestinal processes. Barbiturates are primarily absorbed through the intestine rather than the stomach, but food in the stomach may slow the drug's passage and thus its absorption. Distribution of the various barbiturates depends upon the degree to which they are lipid-soluble. The thiobarbiturates (e.g., thiopental, methohexital) are very lipid-soluble, and their distribution is dependent upon the vascular flow, with areas such as the kidney, liver, and gray matter of the central nervous system quickly reaching maximal levels. The oxybarbiturates (e.g., phenobarbital) approach maximal tissue levels much more slowly (Harvey, 1985).

In general, the barbiturates are eliminated over a period of several days. Thus, repeated administration at the same dose may cause accumulation. This problem is somewhat negated by the increased metabolism seen with chronic dosing, but accumulation must still be considered and dosing adjusted in conjunction with monitoring of blood levels (Harvey, 1985).

Dose and Schedule of Administration. Barbiturates are subject to the Controlled Substances Act of 1970 and are available through prescription, both alone and in combination with other drugs. Most barbiturates are administered orally, but preparations for rectal, subcutaneous, intramuscular, or intravenous administration are also available.

Adjustment to the smallest dose that shows adequate clinical effectiveness is recommended for all drugs in this group. Reduced starting and final dosage levels is suggested in geriatric and dehydrated patients and for patients with poor liver function. The barbiturates used for sedative and hypnotic effect are listed in Table 5.2 along with their trade names and the approximate adult daily dose range. As with the benzodiazepines, barbiturate treatment for insomnia should be of finite duration of from 1 to 3 weeks.

Mechanism of Action. The mechanism of action of barbiturates in the central nervous system appears to be a combination of both postsyn-

Table 5.2. Barbiturates

Barbiturate	Trade Name	Sedative Daily Adult Dose Range (mg/day)	Hypnotic Daily Adult Dose Range (mg/day)
amobarbital	Amytal, Tuinal	30–240	65–200
apobarbital	Alurate	120	40–160
butabarbital	Butisol Sodium, Buticaps, Butalan	45–120	45–100
mephobarbital	Mebaral	96–400	n.a.
methohexital	Brevital	n.a.	50–120
pentobarbital	Nembutal	40–160	100–200
phenobarbital	Solfoton, Barbita, Luminal	30–120	100–320
secobarbital	Seconal, Sodium Pulvules	n.a.	100–200
talbutal	Lotusate	60–180	120

aptic suppression and enhanced inhibition. Inhibition is at least partially mediated by GABA systems, where barbiturates enhance binding. Although barbiturates depress all central nervous system activity, much of the drugs' sedative and hypnotic effects appears concentrated in the reticular activating system. Other brain areas affected include the posterior hypothalamus, the amygdala, and the hippocampus. In the peripheral nervous system, barbiturates reduce activity at autonomic ganglia.

Untoward Effects. Respiration is depressed by barbiturates in a dose-dependent fashion, but in most patients the effect is not clinically significant at up to three times the recommended hypnotic dose. However, patients with pulmonary insufficiency may suffer increased risk of serious respiratory depression even at these relatively low doses. Cardiovascular effects include minor hypotension and decreased heart rate, no more prominent than during normal sleep. Gastrointestinal effects at low doses are also minimal.

Relatively common adverse effects of barbiturates include drowsiness, changes in mood, irritability, impaired judgment, and reduced fine motor skill up to 22 hours after administration (Harvey, 1985). Less common side effects are nausea, vomiting, diarrhea, and dizziness. Sleep disturbance, usually nightmares and rapid eye movement (REM) rebound, may also occur after prolonged use. Barbiturates occasionally cause paradoxical excited states in elderly patients or those in severe pain. Allergic reactions, which are rare, are usually characterized by swellings and inflammation of the skin.

Barbiturate poisoning is a substantial risk, especially with the longer acting forms. The delayed onset of action, along with perceptual time distortion induced by the drugs, may lead to accidental overdose. Acute toxicity symptoms include central nervous system depression, respiratory depression, hypotension, renal failure, hypothermia, coma, and pneumonia (Dimijian, 1984). Lethal doses are approximately 10 times the normal hypnotic dose, or 3.0 grams for short-acting barbiturates and 5.0 grams for the longer-acting drugs. Treatment for overdose is supportive, including respiratory assistance and standard treatment for shock if necessary. If ingestion was recent, activated charcoal administration, gastric lavage, and forced diuresis may be beneficial (McEvoy, 1988).

Physical Dependence. Although barbiturates may be administered for several years without adverse effect, high daily doses can cause physical and psychological dependence. It appears that approximately 700 mg/day (amobarbital, butabarbital, pentobarbital, secobarbital) for 2 months will produce signs of physical dependence (McEvoy, 1988). In addition to the expected effects of barbiturate administration, such as nonanalgesic sedation, slurred speech, and increased emotional response, the symptoms of toxicity include ataxia, double vision, nystagmus, and vertigo. Even though tolerance to some effects of barbiturates occurs after repeated administration, the lethal or acute toxic dose does not appreciably increase with chronic use.

Abstinence and withdrawal from chronic barbiturate use is dangerous and requires careful monitoring. Abstinence symptoms typically appear 8 to 12 hours after the last administration. Symptoms include relatively mild occurrences of nausea, weakness, insomnia, and hypotension and/or more severe symptoms such as delirium and seizures, similar to those seen under severe alcohol withdrawal (McEvoy, 1988). Treatment for barbiturate dependence requires hospitalization and a gradual withdrawal of the drug over several days. Usually, a therapeutic dose of pentobarbital is first administered, and additional doses are added until withdrawal symptoms dissipate. This basal dose level is then decreased daily (40 to 100 mg) over a 7- to 21-day period, depending on severity of dependence. This long withdrawal period reduces the risk of seizures as the drug dose is tapered (Harvey, 1985).

Drug Interactions. CNS depression is potentiated when barbiturates are given concomitantly with other CNS depressants such as alcohol, antihistamines, neuroleptics (see chapter 4), and other sedative–hypnotics. Barbiturates decrease the absorption, and hence the effectiveness, of warfarin sodium and griseofulvin. Barbiturates also appear to increase the metabolism and thus reduce the potency of corticosteroids, antidepressants (see chapter 7), doxycycline, and oral contraceptives. A few drugs, including the monoamine oxidase inhibitors (see chapter 7), are known to inhibit the metabolism of barbiturates and thus increase their half-lives and potentiate their effects. Ketamine anesthesia after barbiturate preoperative administration produces excessive respiratory depression (McEvoy, 1988; Harvey, 1985).

Other Sedatives and Hypnotics

Several drugs besides the benzodiazepines and barbiturates are used as sedatives or hypnotics. Although these drugs are seldom the treatment of choice and may have serious untoward effects or abuse potential, they are nonetheless prescribed in surprising quantities.

Chloral Hydrate. Chloral hydrate is both a hypnotic and a sedative and appears to act similarly to the barbiturates. The drug is supplied as capsules, suppositories, and in solution and is given once daily before bed as a hypnotic or just before surgery as a preoperative sedative. If used as a general sedative, chloral hydrate is usually given 3 times daily in equally divided doses. The most common untoward effects are gastrointestinal and include nausea and diarrhea. Carry-over effects, similar to those of the longer-acting benzodiazepines, may be reported when the drug is used as a hypnotic. Physical and psychological dependence, along with tolerance, may develop with chronic use as brief as 2 weeks (McEvoy, 1988). Overdosage resembles symptoms of alcohol intoxication or barbiturate poisoning. Treatment of overdosage is usually confined to supportive therapy. Chloral hydrate will act additively with all other CNS depressants, including alcohol. Concurrent use of chloral hydrate with furosemide and oral anticoagulants should be avoided.

Ethchlorvynol. Ethchlorvynol (Placidyl) is a hypnotic used for temporary treatment of insomnia. It is available in capsule form for oral ingestion at bedtime. The mechanism of action is unknown. Untoward effects include hypotension, nausea, facial numbness, drowsiness, carry-over fatigue, and nightmares (McEvoy, 1988). Physical and psychological dependence may occur with prolonged use, as may tolerance. Symptoms of dependence are similar to those of the barbiturates. Treatment of physical dependence involves slow withdrawal of the drug, preferably in a hospital setting. Overdosage symptoms are similar to those of the barbiturates and require general supportive therapy. The effects of ethchlorvynol are additive with other CNS depressants. Oral anticoagulants should not be used concurrently with ethchlorvynol. When monoamine inhibitors or some tricyclic antidepressants (see chapter 7) are used concurrently, doses of ethchlorvynol may need to be reduced.

Glutethimide. Glutethimide (Doriden) is used as a hypnotic for temporary relief of insomnia. The drug is not recommended for periods of use longer than 1 week. Glutethimide is available in capsule and tablet form. Although the drug is a CNS depressant, its mechanism of action is unknown. Untoward effects include drowsiness, skin rash, nausea, dry mouth, blurred vision, and diarrhea. Many of these untoward effects are due to its anticholinergic action. Physical and psychological dependence, similar to that associated with the barbiturates, often occurs with prolonged administration of high doses of glutethimide. Treatment for dependence includes gradual withdrawal of the drug with supportive therapy. Overdosage requires general supportive therapy and gastric lavage. Other CNS depressants are additive when used concomitantly with glutethimide. Drugs with anticholinergic action may increase the anticholinergic side effects associated with glutethimide. Concurrent use of oral anticoagulants and glutethimide should be avoided.

Hydroxyzine. Hydroxyzine (Vistaril, Hy-Pam, Hydroxacen, Atarax, Durrax) is an antihistamine used for sedation and as an antianxiety agent. The drug is available in oral solution and suspension and in capsule, tablet, and injectable forms. For anxiety, hydroxyzine is usually divided into four equal doses of from 10 to 25 mg each (50 to 100 mg/day). The drug is a subcortical CNS depressant with anticholinergic, antispasmodic, and local anesthetic properties. Untoward effects are relatively mild at recommended dose levels. The most common complaints involve dry mouth and drowsiness. Overdosage is characterized by excessive sedation and requires general supportive therapy and gastric lavage. Physical dependence does not develop, and the drug is not abused. Hydroxyzine is additive with other central nervous system depressants and may also combine additively with anticholinergic agents to heighten untoward effects. Epinephrine's vasopressor effects will be blocked by hydroxyzine.

Meprobamate. Meprobamate (Equanil, Miltown, Meprospan, Milprem, Deprol, Hepto-M) is a CNS depressant used in the treatment of anxiety. The mechanism of action is unknown. This drug is always administered orally in divided doses (3 or 4 per day) up to a total of 1.0 to 2.0 grams per day. The usual hypnotic dose is approximately 0.8 grams (800 mg) at bedtime. The most predominant untoward effects are drowsiness and impaired muscular coordination *(ataxia)*. Other side effects include dizziness and vertigo, slurred speech, headache, abnormal sensations *(paresthesia)*, euphoria, and weakness (McEvoy, 1988). Mild allergic reactions and paradoxical reactions (e.g., excitement or agitation) sometimes occur. Meprobamate may also adversely affect cardiovascular function (produce palpitation, arrhythmias, hypotension) and may cause nausea and diarrhea. Use of high doses of meprobamate for extended periods may cause physical and psychological dependence. Symptoms of physical dependence are similar to those described for the barbiturates and include drowsiness, ataxia, and dizziness. Withdrawal should be gradual, accompanied by general supportive therapy and close monitoring. Seizures have been known to occur during withdrawal, especially in patients with a previous seizure history or susceptibility. Overdosage symptoms resemble those for barbiturates and require general supportive therapy with special attention to maintenance of respiratory function and adequate blood pressure. Caution should be used when meprobamate is combined with any other central nervous system depressant. Concurrent oral anticoagulant use should be avoided.

Methyprylon. Methyprylon (Noludar) is a CNS depressant, similar to the barbiturates, used as a hypnotic for the short-term treatment of sleep disorders. It is available for oral administration in tablets and capsules. The adult hypnotic dose is 200 to 400 mg per day at bedtime. Sedative doses are also around 300 mg per day in 3 or 4 divided doses. The drug's mechanism of action is unknown. Untoward effects include drowsiness, dizziness, headache, sleep disturbance, gastrointestinal disturbance, and a possible paradoxical reaction (excitation and agitation). High doses for prolonged periods may cause physical dependence, with symptoms of intoxication and withdrawal similar to those of the barbiturates. Withdrawal from methyprylon should be gradual with careful monitoring. Overdosage of methyprylon resembles that of the barbiturates and should be treated similarly, with general supportive therapy and careful monitoring of respiration and cardiovascular activity. Concurrent use of other drugs that suppress the CNS should be carefully managed to avoid excessive sedation.

Diphenhydramine and Bromodiphenhydramine. Diphenhydramine (Alka-Seltzer Plus, Beldin, Benadryl, Benahist, Benoject, Benylin, Compoz, Diphen, Diphenacen, Excedrin P.M., Genahist, Hydramine, Hyrexin, Kapseals, Nervine, Nordryl, Nytol, Sleep-eze, Sleepinal, Sominex, Tusstat, Unisom, Valderine, Wehdryl) and bromodiphenhydramine (Amberyl) are antihistaminic drugs often prescribed and obtained over the counter for their hypnotic actions. These drugs are widely used for maladies as diverse as coughing and Parkinson's disease. As an over-the-counter hypnotic for adults, 50 mg of diphenhydramine is administered orally just before bedtime. The daily dose may be increased under direction of a physician. Treatment should not last for more than 2 weeks. Antihistamines act by blocking the H_1 histamine receptor, thus preventing the endogenous physiological activity of histamine. Histamine acts in several physiological systems including the endocrine, cardiovascular, and extravascular smooth muscle. In general, the toxicity of antihistamines, including diphenhydramine, is low, and they are relatively safe. Their main undesirable effects are related to their anticholinergic activity. Untoward effects can include drowsiness, poor muscle control or weakness, gastrointestinal disturbances, and hypersensitivity reactions. Paradoxical excitation and agitation may also occur. Overdosage usually causes CNS depression in adults, but it may result in central nervous system excitation in children. Treatment of overdosage consists of supportive therapy and may require physostigmine to counteract anticholinergic effects and/or antiepileptic drugs if seizures occur. Diphenhydramine is not typically abused, but its prolonged use as a sleep aid may produce a dependence on the drug for initiation of sleep. As with all hypnotics, concurrent use of other central nervous system depressant drugs (including alcohol) will produce additive effects that should be carefully monitored. Because diphenhydramine is available over the counter, particular attention must be paid to use of this drug by persons who may already be receiving another CNS depressant.

EFFICACY

Insomnia

Insomnia is a diverse and etiologically heterogeneous malady characterized by difficulty in initiating or maintaining sleep and by the feeling that one is not well rested after awakening in the morning. For *difficulty in initiating sleep,* the severity of the condition is a direct function of the time from first retiring to sleep onset. This condition has been associated with aging but may also accompany depression and anxiety. *Early morning awakening,* and subsequent difficulty in returning to sleep, is also associated with aging but may accompany anxiety or depression. Related sleep disorders, usually referred to as *disorders of the sleep–wake schedule,* are characterized by drowsiness and somnolence during the day and disrupted sleep at night. Such a disruption may be associated with CNS damage due to injury or disease or to frequent forced reversals of normal circadian rhythm (e.g., shift work or frequent and rapid time-zone changes) but often involves improper use of the sedative or hypnotic drugs themselves (Crook, Kupfer, Hoch & Reynolds 1987). The prevalence of insomnia disorders is unknown, but at least 15% of the general public occasionally seeks treatment for this condition (American Psychiatric Association, 1987).

In many cases the treatment of choice for insomnia does not involve a drug at all. If the primary problem involves initiation of sleep, phar-

macological therapy may be effective in reducing the latency from retiring to falling asleep, but such a gain must be weighed against the
risks and untoward effects of the drug. An additional half hour of sleep
per night probably does not warrant pharmacological intervention. The
withdrawal from almost all hypnotics usually includes an exacerbation
of the original sleep disturbance. Thus, if the cause of the insomnia is
unchanged, the patient is often worse off after treatment than before.
For situationally specific causes of insomnia, such as jet lag or sleeping
in unfamiliar surroundings, hypnotics may be appropriately prescribed
for a few nights. With more sustained but temporary insomnia, due to
such phenomena as illness or family-related stress, hypnotics may be
efficacious, but should be limited to no more than 2 or 3 weeks of
continuous use. For long-term insomnia, hypnotics should be used for
a maximum of from 3 to 6 months and always in conjunction with
other forms of therapy. In these instances the risk of dependence, tolerance, and severely disrupted sleep patterns is substantial.

An additional group of sleep disorders, called *parasomnias,* involve
the occurrence of an abnormal event during sleep. A recently described
parasomnia called *rapid eye movement sleep behavior disorder (RBD)* is
characterized by the emergence of complex and vigorous movement
during rapid eye movement (REM) sleep (Schenck, Bundlie, Patterson
& Mahowald, 1987). A second sleep disorder of this type, called *periodic
movements of sleep,* formerly called nocturnal myoclonis, is characterized
by repeated, strong, brief contractions of a group of muscles, usually
the lower extremities, during sleep. Both of these parasomnias characteristically respond to treatment with hypnotics, especially the benzodiazepine clonazepam (Klonopin).

As a pharmacological treatment for insomnia, the benzodiazepines
are currently the drugs of choice. They are superior hypnotics compared with the barbiturates and chloral derivatives because they produce fewer side effects, have a greater margin of safety, and a lower
abuse potential. As hypnotics, their main effects on sleep include the
reduction of sleep latency, that is, of the time from first attempt at
sleep to actual sleep onset, a decrease in the number of nighttime
awakenings, and an overall decrease in awake time. Benzodiazepines
are also an effective treatment for "night terrors" (Harvey, 1985), but
they are by no means the treatment of choice for this disorder.

Currently in the United States, three benzodiazepines, flurazepam
(Dalmane), temazepam (Restoril) and triazolam (Halcion), are used primarily as hypnotics. They have marked different half-lives (50 to 100
hours for flurazepam, 10 to 20 hours for temazepam, and 2 to 5 hours
for triazolam) and very different rates of absorption. Flurazepam and
triazolam are rapidly absorbed, and temazepam is slowly absorbed. These

rates of absorption are related to their therapeutic application in that temazepam has shown little efficacy as a treatment for initial insomnia, whereas flurazepam and triazolam are effective in inducing sleep. Flurazepam, which increases total sleep time (Connor, 1984), maintains effectiveness during long-term treatment and shows less severe withdrawal symptoms and less rebound insomnia. The drug is not used extensively today because of its tendency to accumulate over days and to produce significant daytime carry-over sedation, especially during the first few days of treatment. Temazepam is ineffective in inducing sleep because of its slow absorption. The drug is moderately effective in maintaining sleep but shows considerable carry-over of sedative effects into daytime hours (Connor, 1984). Rebound insomnia following abrupt withdrawal may also be a significant problem.

Triazolam is effective in both inducing sleep and maintaining sleep and is perhaps the most often prescribed benzodiazepine for sleep disturbance. As the drug is rapidly eliminated from the body, its carry-over effects are minimal. Tolerance develops rapidly to the therapeutic effects of triazolam, which may necessitate progressive dosage increases. Moreover, some patients experience substantial sleep disturbance, anxiety, and tension during withdrawal (Kales & Kales, 1983).

Although the general effects of the benzodiazepines are very similar, differences in their duration of action and potency have resulted in different therapeutic applications in the treatment of insomnia. Long-acting drugs such as flurazepam, taken as a bedtime hypnotic, may produce sedative effects that intrude on waking hours the next day, causing drowsiness and unwanted decreases in activity. Low doses of a short-acting drug, such as oxazepam (Serax), may be sufficient for daytime reduction of anxiety but inadequate for full coverage as a nighttime hypnotic. Thus, choosing the correct member of the benzodiazepine class for treatment of the various forms of insomnia is of particular importance.

Anxiety

The diagnosis of anxiety reflects an extremely diverse set of causes; its major component, fear, is a ubiquitous phenomenon not always inappropriate or demanding of treatment. Anxiety may occur as a separate condition but is more often regarded as a symptom of other psychiatric disorders (e.g., depression). The condition is characterized by chronic unjustified fear and/or recurring attacks of severe fear or panic. It is most often seen in young adults and more often in women than men. Anxiety often is accompanied by acute panic attacks, characterized by a sudden feeling of extreme fear, choking, hyperventilation, rapid heart beat, palpitations, pain, tremor, sweating, gastrointestinal upset, weakness, dizziness, and nausea (American Psychiatric Association, 1987; Pasnau, 1984). The diagnosis of *panic disorder* may be made when panic attacks recur as a primary symptom of anxiety. Unlike acute panic attacks, which last from a few minutes to 1 or 2 hours, the chronic anxiety symptoms of *generalized anxiety disorder* (American Psychiatric Association, 1987) frequently last from a few days to several months. Chronic anxiety symptoms resemble acute panic attacks but are less severe and are associated with persistent feelings of discomfort and uneasiness.

All drugs of the sedative–hypnotic class appear to exert antianxiety effects, although they differ widely in terms of mechanism of action, duration of effect, potency, side effects, and abuse potential. Their most notable shared pharmacological effect is sedation. Benzodiazepines have generally been proven more effective than barbiturates or meprobamate and currently are the overwhelming choice in the treatment of anxiety. Their popularity as anxiolytics is also due to their lower side-effects profile, which shows less abuse potential, less sedation, and a greater toxicity threshold compared with barbiturates (Rosenbaum, 1982). Because they can produce anterograde amnesia, benzodiazepines are especially useful in treating preoperative fear.

The selection of a particular benzodiazepine to treat anxiety is not based on differences in anxiolytic efficacy (Greenblat, Shader & Abernathy, 1978). In fact, clinical trials show only a few benzodiazepines more effective than a placebo in relieving anxiety at doses that do not cause general nonspecific depression. Even when a drug shows some superiority over a placebo, the difference is often small (Connor, 1984; Lydiard, Roy-Byrne & Ballenger, 1988). Duration of action is perhaps the most relevant information upon which to base the choice of a particular benzodiazepine. Short-acting benzodiazepines (e.g., alprazolam, lorazepam, oxazepam) may be somewhat more appropriate for acute anxiety attacks and p.r.n. (as-needed) administration. Alprazolam has been used effectively with panic disorders and in treating anxiety associated with depression (Sheehan, 1980), but clonazepam appears to be the current drug of choice for these disorders. Chlordiazepoxide and diazepam have traditionally been prescribed for children, but there is no clear rationale for this practice. The benzodiazepines are most effective as a short-term therapy for acute anxiety in patients with a transitory and treatable medical condition or in patients with a primary anxiety diagnosis. These drugs are also prescribed for long-term anxiety disorders. Some of the benzodiazepines, most notably oxazepam, are preferred in the treatment of patients with poor liver function and in the elderly (Baldessarini, 1985b).

Other Disorders

Drugs of the sedative–hypnotic–anxiolytic class are also prescribed for the treatment of epilepsy. This condition and its pharmacological treatment are discussed in chapter 8. Many drugs of the sedative–hypnotic–anxiolytic class are effectively used as an adjunct to other measures in the treatment of skeletal muscle spasticity (increased muscle tone associated with upper motor neuron dysfunction) (Bianchine, 1985). Some movement disorders, such as *myoclonus, chorea, dystonia, tremor,* and the sleep-related movement disorders, may respond favorably to benzodiazepines. *Acute alcohol withdrawal,* and the management of associated symptoms of agitation, tremor, delirium tremens, and hallucinations, may also benefit from benzodiazepine therapy (Ritchie, 1985). Finally, some benzodiazepines, particularly diazepam, are used in the treatment of *neonatal opiate withdrawal* (Jaffee, 1985).

CONCLUDING COMMENT

The drugs considered in this chapter have a wide range of actions. As psychotropic medications, they are useful for inducing sleep, calming agitation, and reducing anxiety. Although these actions can certainly be of significant benefit to patients, it is often possible to manage sleep disorders, agitation, and anxiety through nonpharmacological means. Because of this alternative and the various side effects of the drugs (including a potential for abuse), there has in recent years been a trend towards increased caution in the use of sedatives, hypnotics, and anxiolytics. With some exceptions for cases where benefits are obvious and alternative treatments absent, the long-term use of such medications is difficult to justify.

Chapter 6

Stimulants

The term stimulant has no precise referent, but generally it is applied to drugs that at moderate doses increase subjective arousal and reduce fatigue. As many drugs that produce such actions also increase electrical activity in the CNS and in the sympathetic branch of the peripheral nervous system, they are sometimes termed CNS *stimulants* or *sympathomimetic agents*. Another common designation, *psychomotor stimulants*, emphasizes the fact that agents so categorized may elevate motor activity.

Drugs with dissimilar behavioral and physiological actions (e.g., caffeine, cocaine, nicotine, and strychnine) have been grouped together as stimulants. The majority of stimulants have no psychotherapeutic application, but some are used to treat hyperactivity in children. Medications most often used for this purpose today are methylphenidate (Ritalin), dextroamphetamine (Dexedrine), and pemoline (Cylert). Amphetamine (Benzedrine) was once commonly used but is rarely prescribed today. The effects of amphetamine are essentially identical to those of dextroamphetamine; only the latter agent is discussed in detail here. A fifth stimulant, deanol (Deaner), was occasionally prescribed as a psychotropic medication in the past (e.g., Lewis & Lewis, 1977) but now is almost never used.

HYPERACTIVITY

The term *hyperactivity* is somewhat confusing because it is used both as a diagnostic construct and as a behavioral characteristic. As a behavioral characteristic, hyperactivity refers to overactivity and motor restlessness. As a diagnostic construct, however, hyperactivity is a particular childhood disorder that is defined in a specific way and diagnosed according to certain criteria. Approximate synonyms for hyperactivity in the sense of a diagnostic category are *hyperkinetic reaction of childhood, hyperkinetic syndrome, minimal brain dysfunction,* and *attention-deficit disorder* (with hyperactivity and without hyperactivity). Each of these terms has been somewhat popular. Another designation, *Attention-deficit Hyperactivity Disorder* (ADHD), is employed in the current edition of the *Diagnostic and Statistical Manual of Mental Disorders* (DSM-III-R) of the American Psychiatric Association (1987), but it has not replaced hyperactivity as a diagnostic label, and one currently sees both terms used and defended.

There is no specific diagnostic test for hyperactivity. Table 6.1 lists the defining characteristics of ADHD as described in DSM-III-R. The essential features of the disorder are behaviors that indicate developmentally inappropriate motor restlessness, inattention, and impulsivity. These behaviors appear during the preschool or early school years and are most evident in settings that include peers and require sustained attention and sitting still (e.g., during academic activities). The specific behaviors taken to be indicative of ADHD are age-related. In young children, the usual manifestations involve gross motor activities such as running, an inability to sit still, and frequent shifts from one activity to another.

Older children often appear fidgety and frequently engage in motor activities that appear to be unorganized and not goal-directed. They frequently do not stay on task for appropriate periods of time and may have difficulty in following instructions. Conduct problems (e.g., aggression directed toward peers, defiance of authority figures) are often observed. These and related problems may lead parents and teachers to label the child as unmanageable. School performance is usually poor. There does not, however, appear to be a clear relation between intelligence and ADHD.

It was once believed that children automatically "grew out of" hyperactivity at about the time of puberty. This is not the case. Motor activity often does decrease, but the other problems associated with hyperactivity may persist into adolescence and adulthood (Thorley, 1984). Nonetheless, most of the children diagnosed as hyperactive will lead relatively normal lives as adults. Detailed descriptions of the kinds of behaviors associated with hyperactivity at various ages are provided by Ross and Ross (1982).

Hyperactivity is the most common chronic behavior disorder among preadolescents. Prevalence figures vary across surveys, however, in part because of a lack of precise and objective diagnostic criteria. The generally agreed-upon prevalence among elementary school children is between 5% and 10% (Gadow, 1986a). Hyperkinesis is diagnosed more

Table 6.1. Diagnostic Criteria for Attention-Deficit Hyperactive Disorder

---

Note: Consider a criterion met only if the behavior is considerably more frequent than that of most people of the same mental age.

A. A disturbance of at least six months during which at least eight of the following are present:

    (1) often fidgets with hands or feet or squirms in seat (in adolescents, may be limited to subjective feelings of restlessness)

    (2) has difficulty remaining seated when required to do so

    (3) is easily distracted by extraneous stimuli

    (4) has difficulty awaiting turn in games or group situations

    (5) often blurts out answers to questions before they have been completed

    (6) has difficulty following through on instructions from others (not due to oppositional behavior or failure of comprehension), e.g., fails to finish chores

    (7) has difficulty sustaining attention in tasks or play activities

    (8) often shifts from one uncompleted activity to another

    (9) has difficulty playing quietly

    (10) often talks excessively

    (11) often interrupts or intrudes on others, e.g., butts into other children's games

    (12) often does not seem to listen to what is being said to him or her

    (13) often loses things necessary for tasks or activities at school or at home (e.g., toys, pencils, books, assignments)

    (14) often engages in physically dangerous activities without considering possible consequences (not for the purpose of thrill-seeking), e.g., runs into the street without looking

Note: The above items are listed in descending order of discriminating power based on data from a national field trial of the DSM-III-R criteria for Disruptive Behavior Disorders.

B. Onset before the age of seven.

C. Does not meet the criteria for a Pervasive Developmental Disorder.

Criteria for severity of Attention-deficit Hyperactivity Disorder:

Mild: Few, if any, symptoms in excess of those required to make the diagnosis **and** only minimal or no impairment in school.

Moderate: Symptoms or functional impairment intermediate between "mild" and "severe."

Severe: Many symptoms in excess of those required to make the diagnosis **and** significant and pervasive impairment in functioning at home and school and with peers.

Note: From American Psychiatric Association: *Diagnostic and Statistical Manual of Mental Disorders, Third Edition, Revised,* pp. 52–53. Washington, DC, American Psychiatric Association, 1987. Reprinted by permission.

frequently in boys than in girls; the ratio of male to female cases is at least 4:1. Progress has been made in identifying some of the variables that contribute to hyperactivity, but its etiology is far from being completely understood. There is no single known cause of hyperactivity, although a number of specifiable variables (e.g., maternal alcohol consumption during pregnancy, ingestion of lead during childhood) increase the likelihood of the disorder (Ross & Ross, 1982).

The exact number of children and adolescents who receive stimulant medications is not known, but treatment prevalence surveys show that between 1% and 2% of the total school-age population receives such drugs (Gadow, 1986a). Moreover, most children who receive the diagnosis of ADHD receive stimulant medication at some time. Although this is not widely recognized, approximately 75,000 mentally retarded children and adolescents are currently receiving stimulant medications, primarily for the treatment of hyperactivity. This places stimulants among the behavior-change medications most frequently prescribed for mentally retarded people (Gadow & Poling, 1988).

There is no standard procedure for diagnosing hyperactivity. In research settings and in clinics that specialize in hyperactivity, a battery of assessment instruments is frequently employed. In most other settings, the diagnosis is made on the basis of verbal reports by caregivers and developmental history. There is ongoing debate about the relation of hyperactivity symptoms to other diagnostic categories and about the validity and reliability of the DSM-III-R diagnostic scheme.

HISTORY OF STIMULANT MEDICATIONS

Although it was first synthesized in 1887, amphetamine was not marketed until 1932, when Smith Kline & French offered its "Benzedrine Inhaler" as a decongestant. Three years later, dextroamphetamine (an isomer of amphetamine) was introduced for the treatment of narcolepsy, a rare disorder associated with uncontrollable sleepiness. This treatment remains one of the recognized clinical applications of stimulant medications.

The first report of the efficacy of amphetamine as a psychotropic medication for children was an open clinical trial conducted by Charles Bradley (1937). He reported that about half of a group of 30 elementary school-aged children with behavior and learning problems who received amphetamine in a residential school setting showed a marked therapeutic response. In his words,

> To see a single daily dose of benzedrine produce a greater improvement in school performance than the combined efforts of a capable staff working in a most favorable setting would have been all but demoralizing to teachers, had not the improvement been so gratifying from a practical viewpoint. (p. 582)

Soon after its introduction, amphetamine was observed to reduce hunger in narcoleptic patients. Beginning in the early 1940s, the drug was used widely as a "diet pill," and for many years this was the major clinical application of the amphetamines. It is now recognized that although these drugs are effective in reducing food intake over the short term, they are not useful in long-term weight control.

Many World War II troops used amphetamines to minimize the effects of fatigue. After the war, the Japanese government allowed large stockpiles of methamphetamine to be sold without prescription, and the drug companies marketed them effectively. Abuse became commonplace, and by 1954 the Japanese Pharmacologists Association estimated that about 2% of the population was abusing amphetamine (Ray & Ksir, 1987). By 1960, however, control of production, development of treatment programs, and widespread public education had substantially reduced abuse of amphetamines in Japan.

Easy postwar availability of amphetamines was not confined to Japan, and abuse of these drugs emerged as a problem in many other countries. The problem was not widely recognized in the United States until the 1960s, when intravenous self-administration of "speed" became popular. By 1970, over 10 billion amphetamine tablets were legally manufactured in the United States each year, and Greaves (1980) estimated that in the early 1970s at least 10% of the United States population over 14 years of age had used some form of amphetamine.

Dextroamphetamine, amphetamine, and methamphetamine are currently classified under the Comprehensive Drug Abuse and Control Act of 1970 as Schedule II drugs. Drugs so classified have recognized medical uses, but their abuse potential is high and their production is controlled. Substantial penalties are associated with the illegal manufacturing and distribution of these substances, but the abuse of stimulants continues to be a significant problem in the United States and elsewhere.

Methylphenidate was synthesized in Switzerland in 1954 and soon after appeared in American psychiatric practice. The effectiveness of the drug in controlling hyperactivity was documented in the late 1950s (e.g., Zimmerman & Burgemeister, 1958), and methylphenidate is currently the drug most often prescribed for treating this condition. Because it has substantial abuse potential as well as medical uses, it is classified as a Schedule II drug.

Pemoline was approved by the Food and Drug Administration for use with hyperactive children in 1975. Its effectiveness was first established in studies published in the early 1970s (e.g., Conners, Taylor, Meo, Jurtz & Fournier, 1972). Pemoline has relatively low abuse potential and is therefore classified as a Schedule IV drug.

PHARMACOLOGY

Dextroamphetamine and methylphenidate are similar in chemical structure; pemoline is somewhat different. Nevertheless, the three drugs have generally comparable pharmacological properties. They are orally administered and fairly well absorbed and are distributed throughout the body. They cross the blood–brain barrier with ease. The approximate half-life of methylphenidate is 3 to 4 hours following oral ingestion, that of pemoline is 8 to 12 hours, and that of dextroamphetamine 3 to 7 hours in children and 15 to 20 hours in adults. In most cases, behavioral effects can be observed within 30 minutes after ingesting a stimulant. Treated children typically show their best performance approximately 2 hours after taking medication.

Dextroamphetamine is metabolized through a variety of hepatic pathways, but a substantial proportion of dextroamphetamine molecules are excreted unchanged in urine. Methylphenidate is metabolized in the liver to ritalinic acid; about 80% of the drug is excreted in urine in this form (Franz, 1985). Pemoline is also metabolized in the liver; several metabolites have been isolated, but approximately 50% of pemoline molecules are excreted unchanged in urine.

Dose and Schedule of Administration

Dextroamphetamine is available as both generic and trade name (Dexedrine) products. Dexedrine is manufactured by Smith Kline & French and is available as tablets and as an orange-flavored elixir. It is also produced as sustained-released (Spansule) capsules. Methylphenidate (Ritalin) is also available as generic and trade name (Ritalin) products. CIBA Pharmaceutical Company manufactures standard and sustained-released (Ritalin-SR) tablets. Pemoline (Cylert) tablets are supplied by Abbott Laboratories. Chewable pemoline tablets are available.

Methylphenidate and dextroamphetamine are typically administered in one or two oral doses per day. Although some research suggests that one dose taken in the morning adequately controls behavior through the entire school day, between 60% and 80% of children treated with these drugs receive medication in the morning and at noon (Safer & Krager, 1984). A substantial minority of children also receive these drugs late in the day, and one study found that evening administration of sustained-release dextroamphetamine capsules reduced sleep problems in young hyperactive children (Chatoor, Wells, Conners, Seidel & Shaw, 1983). Stimulants produce insomnia in some patients, however, and this is one reason that dextroamphetamine and methylphenidate usually are not administered late in the day.

Treatment with stimulant medication usually begins with a low dose that is gradually increased until the desired therapeutic response is obtained, side effects become intolerable, or the maximal recommended dose is reached. The initial morning dose of methylphenidate is typically 5 to 10 mg, which is increased by 5 mg at weekly intervals. Most patients receive individual doses of methylphenidate ranging from 5 to 15 mg. Some respond favorably to lower doses and others require higher doses (20–30 mg per dose) for effective behavior management. A few children receive 100 mg of methylphenidate per day, but this should be considered an exceptionally high dose.

Clinical lore suggests that dextroamphetamine is about twice as potent as methylphenidate, but the results of controlled investigations do not support this ratio, and the drugs are often prescribed at comparable doses (Gadow, 1981). When dextroamphetamine is given twice a day, treatment is usually begun at 2.5 or 5 mg per dose (1.25 is recommended for children under 6 years of age), and the dose is incremented by 2.5 mg (per dose) each week. The maximum recommended dosage is 40–60 mg per day; most children can be successfully treated with doses of 7.5 or 15 mg given twice each day.

Pemoline is almost always administered once each day in the morning. Most patients receive 56 to 75 mg/day. The manufacturer's recommended maximum dose is 113 mg/day. Pemoline treatment typically begins at 37.5 mg/day and is incremented by 18.75 mg/day at weekly intervals.

Unless otherwise noted, the doses we have described are typical of those used with individuals over 6 years of age; smaller doses are characteristically used with younger children. Although it is common clinical practice to specify stimulant dosage in terms of total amount of drug administered per day or per dose, these designations are imprecise because patients vary in body weight. Even when differences in body weight are accounted for, however, there are sizeable differences in the response of individual patients to the same stimulant dose. Moreover, even within the same individual the nature of the dose–response relationship depends upon the behavior measured. Both of these effects are evident in a study conducted by Sprague and Sleator (1977).

Those investigators examined the heart rate, general classroom behavior, and learning (in a laboratory setting) of 20 hyperactive children under conditions where placebo, 0.3 mg/kg methylphenidate, and 1.0 mg/kg methylphenidate were administered. General classroom behavior (i.e., social behavior) was quantified through the use of the Abbreviated Conners' Teachers Rating Scale (Conners, 1973), and learning was evaluated through the use of a short-term memory task. This task required the child to look briefly at a matrix of children's pictures, then to indicate a few seconds later whether or not a test picture was presented as part of the matrix.

Summary results for the patients as a group are shown in Figure 6.1. Group performance on the short-term memory task was best at 0.3

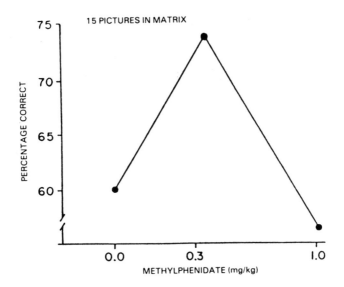

FIGURE 6.1. Effects of two doses of methylphenidate on heart rate, teacher rating of classroom behavior, and learning in a short-term memory task. The data depicted are group averages. *Note:* From "Methylphenidate in Hyperkinetic Children: Differences in Dose Effects on Learning and Social Behavior" by R. L. Sprague and E. K. Sleator, 1977, *Science, 198,* p. 1275. Copyright 1977 by the American Association for the Advancement of Science. Reprinted by permission.

mg/kg, whereas social behavior was best at 1.0 mg/kg. Average heart rate was similar under placebo and 0.3 mg/kg conditions but was considerably elevated at 1.0 mg/kg. These relations did not hold for all patients, however. For example, some children did best in the memory task at 1.0 mg/kg, and others received the best ratings of social behavior at 0.3 mg/kg. These and many other data show that there is no one best stimulant dose for all patients and problems. Consequently, careful consideration must be given to selection of treatment objectives and individualization of dosage for all patients. The goal in individualizing dosage is to find a dose that adequately controls target behaviors without impairing adaptive behavior or inducing serious physiological side effects. Because the likelihood of adverse reactions generally increases with dosage, the lowest dose that adequately controls target behaviors is to be preferred. It must be recognized, however, that insufficient dosage can lead to treatment failure: The patient's response to medication, not the amount given per se, should govern the treatment regimen.

The length of time hyperactive children are exposed to stimulant medication varies enormously across patients. Some children receive a stimulant for a few months, whereas others require pharmacotherapy either continuously or intermittently for many years. Because there is no way to tell if medication is necessary other than by a temporary cessation of treatment, drug-free periods are a critical aspect of follow-up care.

Mechanism of Action

The actions of amphetamines in the central nervous system have been explored extensively. Dextroamphetamine appears to exert most of its effects by releasing catecholamine neurotransmitters (norepinephrine, dopamine) from their storage sites in nerve terminals, which leads to synaptic stimulation. These effects can be blocked by agents that inhibit the synthesis of catecholamines (e.g., methyparatyrosine) but not by agents that interfere with the storage of catecholamines (e.g., reserpine). This distinction suggests that the actions of dextroamphetamine are mediated through a newly synthesized fraction of brain catecholamines (Goth, 1985). In addition to releasing catecholamines, dextroamphetamine interferes with the re-uptake of these neurotransmitters and, at high doses, releases serotonin (a neurotransmitter). Methylphenidate also interacts with catecholaminergic neurons in a manner that leads to synaptic stimulation. It appears to act through a different mechanism, however, because the CNS effects of methylphenidate are blocked by reserpine but not by methylparatyrosine. This suggests that the effects of methylphenidate are mediated through a stored fraction of brain catecholamines.

The neuropharmacological mechanisms of action of pemoline are not known. It is reasonable to assume, but by no means certain, that they are similar to those of dextroamphetamine and methylphenidate.

The therapeutic effects of stimulants cannot be explained in terms of simple behavioral mechanisms of action. One interesting characteristic of these drugs is that their effects are in many cases *rate dependent:* They increase low-rate responses at doses that decrease high-rate responses. This action demonstrates that (a) stimulants do not inevitably increase responding and (b) whether or not they do so is determined in part by the nature of the response. An explanation of the therapeutic response to stimulants in terms of rate dependency does not, however, appear plausible.

Tolerance and Physical Dependence

Substantial tolerance develops to the anorectic and euphoric effects of stimulants. As discussed subsequently, tolerance also develops to many of the side effects of these agents. When stimulants are used in the treatment of hyperactivity, tolerance to therapeutic effects is generally not a problem, even though clinical lore suggests otherwise.

Abrupt discontinuation of chronic stimulant administration does not result in major, grossly observable changes in physiology or behavior. Therefore, it was once assumed that these drugs did not produce physical dependence. Studies of stimulant abusers have made it clear, however, that physical dependence does occur with chronic, high-dose administration of dextroamphetamine and related drugs. It is characterized by signs and symptoms of withdrawal that include hyperphagia (increased food consumption), lethargy, depression, REM sleep rebound, prolonged sleep, general fatigue, and craving for the drug. Significant physical dependence appears to occur rarely if ever when stimulants are used to treat hyperactivity.

EFFICACY

Dozens of articles assessing the effects of stimulants in hyperactive children have been published; several good reviews of stimulant drug therapy are available (e.g., Barkley, 1981; Cantwell & Carlson, 1978; Gadow, 1986a; Ross & Ross, 1982; Whalen, 1982). A relatively large number of tests, rating scales, and direct-observation procedures have been used to evaluate response to stimulant medication, and it is now clear that the effects of these drugs depend in part on the target behaviors selected and the manner in which they are measured.

Laboratory procedures demonstrate that stimulants can in some situations increase the ability to focus and sustain attention, to learn, to inhibit impulses, and to respond promptly and accurately. Clinical data show that stimulants produce a positive therapeutic response in the general deportment of most hyperactive children. As noted by Ross and Ross (1982):

> There is empirical support for a generalized overall improvement in cognitive and behavior symptoms in about two-thirds (Kinsbourne & Swanson, 1979) to three-quarters (Barkley, 1977) of the hyperactive children who are given a trial of stimulant medication. Clinicians usually set the positive response level at about 70 percent with the qualification that allowance must be made for idiosyncratic specificity, that is, the fact that many children will respond well, but not to the first stimulant or psychoactive drug administered (Knopp et al., 1973; Weiss, 1975). (p. 188)

Teachers' ratings, quantified through the use of standardized scales, are among the most used measures of the therapeutic response to stimulant medication. One popular scale is the Abbreviated Teacher Rating Scale (ATRS) (Conners, 1973), which emphasizes classroom behaviors that may be disruptive and yields a composite score ranging from 0 to 30.

Numerous studies in which outcomes were quantified through the ATRS, other rating scales, or global impressions show that most, but not all, hyperactive children exposed to stimulant medication are rated as improved overall. They also typically are judged to be more cooperative, attentive, and compliant when treated with stimulants (Conners & Werry, 1979). Medication also appears to reduce peer-directed aggression in most cases (Gadow et al., in press) and to improve classroom and play behavior as indexed by direct observation (Abikoff, 1982; Whalen, Henker, Collins, Finck & Dotemoto, 1979). Within the therapeutic dosage range, scores on the ATRS and similar scales usually decline with increasing dosage. Such a relation is evident in Figure 6.2, which shows behavioral response to three different doses of methylphenidate.

Stimulant-induced reductions in undesirable behavior, coupled with increases in attention and compliance, make it easier and more pleasant for parents and teachers to deal with the patient. A typical response when parents are asked how their child differs when on medication is that, "He's a lot easier to like. He isn't so fidgety and irritable, and he listens better to what I say." Not surprisingly, improved par-

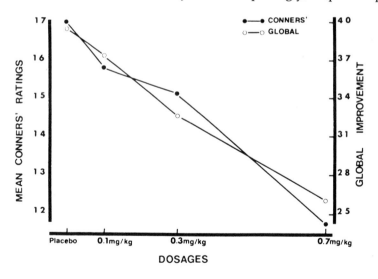

FIGURE 6.2. Effects of three doses of methylphenidate on mean ratings of behavior by teachers employing two different scales. With both scales, classroom behavior improves as scores decrease. *Note:* From "Methylphenidate in the Treatment of Hyperkinetic Children" by E. K. Sleator and A. W. von Neumann, 1974, *Clinical Pediatrics, 13*, p. 23. Copyright 1974 by J. B. Lippincott Company. Reprinted by permission.

ent–child and teacher–child interactions have been reported with stimulant treatment (e.g., Barkley, Karlsson, Strzelecki & Murphy, 1984; Campbell, Endman & Bernfeld, 1977). Interactions with peers often improve as a function of stimulant medication, but this does not happen in all cases (Pelham & Bender, 1982). As Pelham and Murphy (1986) suggest, both medication and social skills training are probably needed to normalize peer relations in some hyperactive children.

The effects of stimulants on academic performance (reviewed by Gadow, 1985, 1986) are difficult to summarize. Several early articles reported that parents and teachers considered increased academic productivity to be a major virtue of stimulant therapy. Investigations in which academic achievement was actually measured did not, however, support this conclusion. Barkley and Cunningham (1978), for example, reviewed the results of 17 short-term and 6 follow-up studies and found little evidence that stimulants generally improved academic achievement. The Barkley and Cunningham review was quite influential, and for several years most experts concluded that stimulants do not typically improve academic performance. However, some recent studies (e.g., Pelham, Bender, Caddell, Booth & Moorer, 1985; Rapport, Murphy & Bailey, 1982; Rapport, Stoner, Du Paul, Birmingham & Tucker, 1985) have confirmed earlier studies (e.g., Bradley & Bowen, 1941) showing that certain hyperactive children complete more schoolwork and learn more when they are medicated than when they are off stimulants. Further investigation of the effects of stimulants on academic performance and achievement is necessary, but it is obvious that medication alone will not produce optimal academic achievement, particularly for hyperactive children who are also learning disabled.

It is sometimes asserted that stimulants are ineffective with mentally retarded children. The limited data available suggest that they are about as effective in the treatment of hyperactivity in mildly to moderately mentally retarded individuals as in other people (Gadow & Poling, 1988).

Although most research has been done with children between 6 and 12 years of age, stimulant medications are used to treat patients from infancy to adulthood, and their effects are not obviously age-related. It has been reported, however, that young children may exhibit (a) a lesser therapeutic response, (b) a more variable therapeutic response, and (c) a greater sensitivity to overmedication (Gadow, 1986).

The therapeutic effects of dextroamphetamine, methylphenidate, and pemoline are similar. Pemoline has been studied much less than the other agents, but it appears to be slightly less effective than dextroamphetamine and methylphenidate (Cantwell & Carlson, 1978; Dykman, McGrew & Ackerman, 1974). Although some patients respond differently to them, it is not possible to predict whether dextroamphetamine, methylphenidate, or pemoline will be most effective for a given patient. Nor is it possible to predict accurately whether a child diagnosed as hyperactive will respond positively to any medication. Unless there is good reason to do otherwise, most physicians prefer an initial trial with methylphenidate, followed by pemoline or dextroamphetamine if necessary.

Stimulant therapy often is effective in reducing the undesired behaviors associated with hyperactivity. Nonetheless, it is limited in at least four respects (Pelham & Murphy, 1986). First, stimulant therapy alone is often not enough to bring children into the normal range of social and academic functioning. Although a child's behavior may improve substantially when medication is administered, the need for psychological and educational interventions will remain. Second, not all hyperactive children respond favorably to stimulant medication. Approximately 70% to 80% of hyperactive children exhibit a clinically meaningful therapeutic response to these drugs. The remainder show little response or an adverse reaction. Moreover, some children experience intolerable behavioral or physiological side effects that prevent their receiving medication at a dosage adequate to control target behaviors. Third, to minimize adverse reactions (e.g., insomnia, anorexia), stimulant medication is often prescribed so that behavior is controlled only during the hours that school is in session. Parents therefore must utilize nonpharmacological interventions to manage their child at home. Unfortunately, these techniques are often of limited value for many parents (for a variety of reasons), who are left with the problem of an unmanageable hyperactive child.

Fourth, the benefits derived from long-term treatment with stimulants are of questionable consequence. Pelham and Murphy (1986) note that

> without exception studies that have followed children treated with psychostimulant medication for periods up to 5 years have failed to provide any evidence that the drugs improve ADD children's long-term prognosis (Charles & Schain, 1981; Riddle & Rapoport, 1976; Satterfield et al., 1982; Weiss et al., 1975). Although their methodology requires that these studies be interpreted cautiously (Pelham, 1983), nonetheless, despite the evidence of short-term gains, beneficial treatment effects do not appear to be maintained when psychostimulant medication, as typically administered, is used as a long-term treatment for the average ADD child. (p. 113)

Stimulant drugs are occasionally described as "chemical straitjackets" that produce children who behave like entranced zombies, perseverating in activities without reason or affect. Surely a medication that produced such actions would be undesirable, but the chemical straitjacket criticism appears to be largely unwarranted. It may have arisen from cases where unduly high doses were prescribed, perhaps combined with a general opposition to pharmacological treatment of behavior problems. Gittelman-Klein (1975a) and others have argued that, far from creating zombies, stimulants if effective actually increase the freedom of hyperactive children because, when they are medicated, control is by appropriate environmental events, not by irrelevant stimuli.

Some researchers have claimed that the actions of stimulants in hyperkinetic children are unique or that the calming effects of stimulants in hyperactive children are "paradoxical." Research suggests, however, that the effects of dextroamphetamine in nonhyperactive boys and normal men (Rapoport, Buchsbaum, Zahn, Weingartner, Ludlow & Mikkelson, 1978; Rapoport, Buchsbaum, Weingartner, Zahan & Ludlow, 1980) are similar to those observed in hyperactive children. Moreover, it is well established that, despite their name, stimulants can (depending upon dose and the response in question) increase, decrease, or have no effect on behavior. Hence the reduction in undesired behaviors (calming) observed in hyperkinetic children is but one example of many "paradoxical" responses to stimulants.

DRUG INTERACTIONS

Children on medication for hyperactivity typically receive a single drug for that condition, although individuals whose behavior is especially difficult to manage may receive combinations of psychotropic medications. Methylphenidate, for example, is sometimes used in combination with imipramine or thioridazine. The latter has been reported to enhance the efficacy of methylphenidate, but this finding should be regarded as tentative (Gittelman-Klein et al., 1976).

Methylphenidate may decrease the effectiveness of certain antihypertensive medications (e.g., guanethidine). The drug increases the response to coumarin anticoagulants, some anticonvulsants (phenytoin, primidone, phenobarbital), and tricyclic antidepressants. Monoamine oxidase (MAO) inhibitors may potentiate cardiovascular and other responses to methylphenidate.

Because dextroamphetamine is a weak base, drugs that increase gastrointestinal acidity (e.g., reserpine) lower its absorption, whereas agents that acidify urine increase its excretion. The result in both cases is a reduction in blood levels and efficacy. The efficacy of dextroamphetamine is increased by drugs that decrease gastrointestinal acidity (e.g., acetazolamide, some thiazides) or urinary acidity.

Dextroamphetamine enhances the action of tricyclic antidepressants;

when it is combined with desipramine or imipramine, cardiovascular effects may be potentiated. MAO inhibitors in combination with dextroamphetamine may lead to a dangerous hypertensive crisis. Chlorpromazine, haloperidol, and other neuroleptics reduce the central nervous systems effects of dextroamphetamine, and lithium carbonate also inhibits its actions. Dextroamphetamine may reduce the absorption and/or slow the metabolism of certain antiepileptic medications (e.g., phenobarbital, phenytoin, ethosuximide). It also increases the analgesic actions of some opioids and reduces the efficacy of antihypertensives.

UNTOWARD EFFECTS

The side effects of dextroamphetamine, methylphenidate, and pemoline are similar, although pemoline has weaker cardiovascular and sympathomimetic actions than the other agents. These drugs at moderate doses rarely produce serious adverse reactions. Two relatively common short-term effects are insomnia and loss of appetite. The former problem can be minimized by administering medication only in the morning (although this regimen will not result in effective behavior control in all patients) or countered by administering a hypnotic agent in the evening. Anorexia can be managed by administering medication just before meals. Less prevalent short-term side effects include headache, stomachache, constipation, diarrhea, dryness of the mouth, skin rashes, irritability, increased talkativeness, drowsiness, changes in mood, and nausea. Tolerance often develops to these effects. To reduce patient discomfort, the dose may in some cases have to be reduced and then gradually increased.

Dextroamphetamine and to a lesser extent methylphenidate can increase heart rate and blood pressure and may produce cardiac arrythmias. These reactions are typically dose-dependent. At therapeutic dosages, increases in heart rate and blood pressure are minimal and do not appear to pose a danger for patients with normal cardiovascular function.

Involuntary movements of the muscles (e.g., grimacing, facial tics, jerking and writhing movements of arms and legs, twisting of the head and neck), Tourette syndrome, glaucoma, and increases in stereotypies or tics have occasionally been reported in patients treated with stimulants. These reactions are rare. Stimulants may precipitate seizures in some patients. This is uncommon, however, and stimulants are used effectively with many children who also receive pharmacotherapy for seizure disorders.

Long-term side effects of stimulant drug therapy have been studied less extensively than short-term effects. The only long-term side effect that has been convincingly documented is reduced rate of growth. Children who receive dextroamphetamine or relatively high doses of methylphenidate gain less height and weight than would be expected had they not received medication. This effect has not been observed with children receiving low to moderate doses of methylphenidate with breaks from medication whenever feasible. Even when stimulants suppress growth rates, an increase in growth rate following the termination of treatment usually compensates for the slower rate while on medication.

Especially when used at high doses, stimulants may lead to undue perseveration, impair cognitive function, or interfere with the performance of adaptive behaviors. These reactions appear to be rare. Other uncommon but serious adverse reactions are hallucinations and psychosis. As the stimulants have substantial potential for abuse, care must be taken that patients do not increase dosage on their own initiative. Receiving stimulant medication during childhood does not appear to increase the likelihood of concurrent or subsequent drug abuse.

Hepatic (liver) dysfunction involving elevated liver enzymes, hepatitis, and jaundice has been reported in patients taking pemoline.

Acute overdosage is rarely a problem when stimulants are used to treat hyperactivity. When it does occur, symptoms reflect overactivation of the CNS and the sympathetic branch of the peripheral nervous system. They may include vomiting, agitation, tremors, hyperreflexia, convulsions, euphoria, muscle twitching, confusion, hallucinations, delirium, sweating, increased body temperature, flushing, increased heart rate, hypertension, drying of mucous membranes, and headache. These reactions may be serious but are rarely fatal if supportive treatment is arranged. In providing such treatment, (a) conditions are arranged so that self-injury is prevented and excitement is minimized, (b) procedures are employed to ensure adequate circulation and respiratory exchange and to reduce blood pressure if seriously elevated, and (c) gastric lavage is used to remove unabsorbed drug from the body. Chlorpromazine antagonizes some of the actions of stimulants and is often administered. Drugs that acidify the urine (e.g., ammonium chloride) speed the excretion of dextroamphetamine and are used therapeutically for this purpose.

A psychotic reaction that closely resembles schizophrenia has been observed in stimulant abusers who take the drugs chronically at high doses. This reaction does not occur at therapeutic doses.

Use of dextroamphetamine is contraindicated in patients with known hypersensitivity, cardiovascular disease, moderate to severe hypertension, hyperthyroidism, or glaucoma. The drug also should not be used with agitated patients or those with a history of drug abuse. Contraindications to methylphenidate are anxiety, glaucoma, motor tics, and hypersensitivity. Some clinicians consider a diagnosis or family history of Tourette syndrome a contraindication, but this is controversial. Pemoline should not be used with patients hypersensitive to the drug or with individuals whose hepatic function is impaired.

There is no standard procedure for detecting side effects of stimulant medication. Direct observation and patient report are the usual means of detecting untoward responses to these drugs. Blood pressure should be periodically monitored in patients receiving stimulant medications, and hepatic function should be assessed in those exposed to pemoline.

ALTERNATIVE AND COLLATERAL TREATMENT

Controlled investigations have shown that systematic behavior modification procedures based on the principles of operant conditioning can be effective in improving the behavior of hyperactive children (O'Leary, 1980; Ross & Ross, 1982). Despite this, such interventions are used rather infrequently. In one survey, behavior therapy had been employed with only 10% of children assigned the diagnosis of attention deficiency disorder, whereas medication had been employed with over 80% (Bosco & Robin, 1980). Studies comparing the effects of behavioral and pharmacological interventions fail to indicate clear superiority for either therapeutic modality. In fact, it is probably impossible to compare meaningfully two therapies so broad in scope. As Mash and Dalby (1979) put it,

> Medication is not a unitary treatment and behavior therapy is even more diverse. What is needed are empirical statements re the effectiveness and/ or relative effectiveness of specific medication regimens or specific behavior therapy interventions, for specific children, with specific behaviors, in specific situations. (p. 217)

Such empirical statements cannot be accurately made at present. It can, however, be asserted with confidence that behavioral interventions can be profitably combined with stimulant therapy. A recent review of studies in which combined pharmacological and behavioral interventions were evaluated (Pelham & Murphy, 1986) found that 13 of 19 independent studies (68%) demonstrated superiority for the combined treatment on at least one outcome measure. Unfortunately, a total of only 167 children participated in these studies, the median duration of treatment was less than 3 weeks, and methodological weaknesses were evident in most of the studies; thus conclusions must be drawn with caution.

Feingold (1974) claimed that 30% to 50% of hyperactive children would exhibit marked behavioral improvement if exposed to a special diet (termed the Feingold or Kaiser-Permanente) that eliminates artificial colors, the preservative butylated hydroxytoluene, and foods that contain salicylates (e.g., raspberries, tomatoes, cucumbers). Despite the claims of Feingold and other advocates, controlled investigations reveal that this diet is not effective for most hyperactive children (Conners, 1980; Prinz, 1985).

Treatment with megavitamins has also been advocated (Cott, 1972), but it is without demonstrated general efficacy (Haslam, Dalby & Rademaker, 1984). Some investigations have shown that caffeine is of value in treating hyperactive children, but results of other studies are contradictory; thus caffeine, too, must be considered a treatment of uncertain worth (Ross & Ross, 1982).

CONCLUDING COMMENT

The primary use of stimulant medications is in treating hyperkinesis in children and adolescents. Stimulants are relatively safe when used therapeutically, and most hyperkinetic patients evidence some degree of therapeutic response to them. Nonetheless, the widespread use of stimulants is controversial, in part because alternatives are available and also because medication alone is unlikely to solve all of the behavioral problems characteristic of hyperkinetic patients. As a rule, stimulant medication should be incorporated as part of an integrated treatment package, and the contribution of the stimulant to that package should be evaluated on a patient-by-patient basis.

Chapter 7
Antidepressants and Lithium

ANTIDEPRESSANTS

The antidepressants consist of several classes of drugs. The most widely used are the tricyclic antidepressants, so named because of their three-ring molecular structure. The first of these compounds, imipramine, was synthesized in the late 1940s. It was very similar in chemical structure to the phenothiazine neuroleptics but, unlike these drugs, was not found to be of clinical value for the treatment of psychosis. It did, however, produce dramatic benefit for certain depressed patients (Kuhn, 1958). Several tricyclics including imipramine are currently approved for use in the United States (see Table 7.1). For the most part, they produce similar therapeutic effects, at least with regard to depression, but their side-effect profiles differ. For example, desipramine (Norpramin, Pertofrane) has less pronounced anticholinergic effects than imipramine and therefore may be preferred with patients whose symptom complex includes somatic complaints.

The oldest class of antidepressant drugs is the MAO inhibitors, three of which are currently approved in the United States for the treatment of depression (see Table 7.1). Tranylcypromine and phenelzine are the most commonly prescribed whereas isocarboxazid is rarely used. Tranylcypromine is structurally similar to amphetamine. The first MAO inhibitor, iproniazid (Marsilid), was developed in the early 1950s and used as an antibacterial agent in the treatment of tuberculosis. It was soon found to have mood-elevating properties, and studies of psychiatric patients revealed its value as an important therapeutic agent for the treatment of depression (Crane, 1959; Kline, 1958). However, iproniazid was later withdrawn from the market as an antidepressant because of toxicity. Unfortunately, the MAO inhibitors produce a potentially fatal toxic reaction when taken in combination with certain

Table 7.1. Antidepressant Drugs and Doses (milligrams per day)

Agent	Brand Names	Usual Dose (mg/d)	Extreme Dose[a] (mg/d)
Tricyclic agents			
Amitriptyline	Amitril, Elavil, Endep (and generic)	100–200	25–600
Amoxapine	Asendin	200–300	50–600
Clomipramine	Anafranil	100–150	25–250
Desipramine	Norpramin, Pertofrane	***	***
Doxepin	Adapin, Sinequan	100–200	25–300
Imipramine	Janimine, SK-Pramine, Tofranil (and generic)	100–200	25–300
Maprotiline	Ludiomil	100–150	25–225[b]
Nortriptyline	Aventyl, Pamelor	75–150	20–150
Protriptyline	Vivactil	15–40	10–60
Trimipramine	Surmontil	75–250	23–300
MAO inhibitors			
Phenelzine	Nardil	45–75	15–90
Tranylcypromine	Parnate	20–30	10–60
Isocarboxazid	Marplan	20–30	10–30
Atypical agents			
Bupropion	Wellbutrin	200–300	100–450
Fluoxetine	Prozac	20–40	10–80
Trazodone	Desyrel (and generic)	150–200	50–600

Note: Adapted from "Current Status of Antidepressants: Clinical Pharmacology and Therapy" by R. J. Baldessarini, 1989, *Journal of Clinical Psychiatry, 50,* p. 118. Copyright 1989 by Physicians Postgraduate Press, Inc. Adapted by permission.
[a] Low extreme doses are for very young or elderly patients (except for imipramine, desipramine, and nortriptyline, reported experience with antidepressants in children is limited); high doses are best reserved for hospitalized patients when low doses are not adequate.
[b] Maprotiline should be used very cautiously in doses above 200 mg/d because of the risk of seizures.

foods and for this reason are generally prescribed only for patients who fail to respond satisfactorily to more conventional drugs. In recent years there has been a renewed interest in the MAO inhibitors because of reports of greater efficacy (when administered in higher doses) and wider clinical application. There are several newer MAO inhibitors not currently approved for general use that may prove to be as effective as standard products but less toxic (Baldessarini, 1989).

The newer antidepressants that differ in chemical structure from the tricyclics and the MAO inhibitors are simply referred to as atypical antidepressants. They include compounds such as the tetracyclic maprotiline (Ludiomil), which is structurally similar to the tricyclics; trazodone (Desyrel); buproprion (Wellbutrin); and fluoxetine (Prozac). A number of other antidepressants are currently under investigation for safety and efficacy (see Baldessarini, 1989).

Pharmacology

The tricyclics are readily absorbed from the intestine, but at high doses the anticholinergic effects of these drugs may actually slow absorption. Peak plasma levels are typically achieved in 2 to 8 hours. Once in the bloodstream, they are highly bound to plasma proteins. In adults, for example, imipramine is approximately 86% bound. The values are lower for young children and the elderly, and subsequently they may experience toxicity at mg/kg doses considered safe for adults. The tricyclics are extensively metabolized by liver enzymes, and some of the metabolites are psychoactive. For example, desipramine and nortriptyline are active metabolites of imipramine and amitriptyline metabolism, respectively. There is considerable between-patient variation in rates of drug metabolism. Tricyclics are metabolized more rapidly by children and more slowly by elderly patients. With the exception of protriptyline, which has a half-life of approximately 60 hours, the tricyclics are completely eliminated from the body within a week after the withdrawal of medication.

The MAO inhibitors are readily absorbed from the gastrointestinal tract. Their maximal enzyme-inhibiting effect is achieved in a few days, but improvement in depressive symptoms may not be present for 2 to 3 weeks. The MAO inhibitors are metabolized by liver enzymes, the rate of which is influenced by genetic factors. Approximately one-half of the European and North American population are slow metabolizers of phenelzine. The percentage is even higher for certain Oriental populations. Following phenelzine withdrawal, it may take the body up to 2 weeks to restore normal levels of MAO. Enzyme recovery is more rapid with tranylcypromine.

Mechanism of Action

Tricyclics are believed to produce their antidepressant action by blocking the re-uptake of certain neurotransmitters (e.g., norepinephrine, serotonin) into the presynaptic membrane, thus increasing neurotransmitter effectiveness by making larger amounts available to receptor sites on the postsynaptic membrane (reviewed by Baldessarini, 1989). Some tricyclics appear to have greater affinity for specific neurotransmitters. For example, desipramine and the tetracyclic maprotiline show relative specificity for norepinephrine, whereas clomipramine has a relatively specific effect on serotonin as do some of the atypical antidepressants (e.g., fluoxetine, trazodone).

The tricyclics also interfere with the actions of the neurotransmitter acetylcholine (and hence are said to be *anticholinergic*), which is present in the brain, the autonomic nervous system, and neurons in the skeletal muscles. These anticholinergic effects explain many of the adverse reactions associated with these drugs. There is considerable variation between tricyclics in their ability to affect acetylcholine receptors. On a scale ranging from most to least anticholinergic, amitriptyline is at the top, imipramine in the middle, and desipramine at the bottom (see Table 7.2). The tetracyclics are less anticholinergic than the tricyclics. Some of the atypical antidepressants (e.g., fluoxetine, trazodone) have virtually no anticholinergic activity.

The tricyclics' ability to interfere with the actions of norepinephrine in sympathetic nervous system neurons may explain their ability to suppress nocturnal enuresis. In addition to being able to potentiate norepinephrine activity, the tricyclics also block a specific type of norepinephrine receptor. Consequently, another possible mechanism for their antienuretic properties is the inhibition of the bladder neck response to norepinephrine.

The primary mode of action of the MAO inhibitors is the irreversible inactivation of the enzyme monoamine oxidase, which is present in the mitochondria. Mitochondria, which are organelles (little organs) found

Table 7.2. Side Effects of Non-MAOI Antidepressants

Antidepressant	Sedation	Insomnia	Anticholinergic Effects	Orthostatic Hypotension	Nausea
Amitriptyline (Elavil and others)	+ + +	0	+ + +	+ + +	0
Amoxapine (Asendin)	+	+ +	+	+ +	0
Desipramine (Norpramin, Pertofrane)	+	0	+	+ +	0
Doxepin (Adapin, Sinequan)	+ + +	0	+ +	+ + +	0
Fluoxetine (Prozac)	+	+ + +	0	0	+ +
Imipramine (Tofranil and others)	+ +	0	+ +	+ + +	0
Maprotiline (Ludiomil)	+ +	0	+ +	+ +	0
Nortriptyline (Pamelor and others)	+ +	0	+	+	0
Protriptyline (Vivactil)	+	+ +	+ + +	+ +	0
Trazodone (Desyrel and others)	+ + +	0	0	+ + +	+
Trimipramine (Surmontil)	+ + +	0	+ + +	+ + +	0

Source: Alan J. Gelenberg, M.D., distillation of literature and clinical impressions.
Symbols: + + + = most
      + + = intermediate
      + = minimal
      0 = none
Note: From "New Perspectives on the Use of Tricyclic Antidepressants" by A. J. Galenberg, 1989, Journal of Clinical Psychiatry, 50, p. 3. Copyright 1989 by Physicians Postgraduate Press, Inc. Reprinted by permission.

in all body cells, generate energy for the cell through the oxidation of foodstuffs. MAO also breaks down various neurotransmitters (e.g., norepinephrine, dopamine, serotonin) in the presynaptic membrane and thereby prevents an excessive accumulation of these substances. When MAO activity is blocked, neurotransmitters accumulate; consequently, more are available for release into the synaptic cleft. These drugs inhibit MAO not only in the mitochondria located in the presynaptic membrane of nerve cells, but in the cells of other organs as well, including the liver. This can interfere with the liver's ability to metabolize substances in the blood, including other drugs. The MAO inhibitors also affect enzymes other than monoamine oxidase, which adds to their toxicity.

Dose and Schedule

General dosage guidelines for the tricyclics are presented in Table 7.1. These guidelines pertain primarily to the treatment of mood disorders. Optimal therapeutic doses for other disorders (e.g., enuresis, migraine headaches, panic disorders) are somewhat lower. Injectable forms of imipramine and amitriptyline are available, but they are used infrequently. Oral preparations of nortriptyline and doxepin can be obtained in both solid and liquid form. Because the tricyclics have relatively long half-lives, patients can be gradually switched from divided daily doses to a single bedtime dose.

Because therapeutic response in depressed patients correlates fairly well with drug blood level, blood assays have become a routine part of clinical management. The approximate therapeutic ranges for three tricyclics are as follows: imipramine (150 to 300 ng/mL), desipramine (125 to 300 ng/mL), nortriptyline (50 to 150 ng/mL), and amitriptyline (150 to 300 ng/mL). The expression ng/mL refers to nanograms per milliliter of blood plasma. (A *nanogram* is one-millionth of a milligram.) Blood level analyses are even more important for preventing toxic reactions due to abnormally high drug blood levels (Preskorn, 1989). Elevated drug blood levels can occur for a variety of reasons, one of which is genetic. Some patients are just slow metabolizers of these drugs. Blood samples should be drawn after the patient has been on a stable dose for 1 week, preferably 12 hours after the last dose taken.

Tolerance and Physical Dependence

Most patients develop a tolerance for the unwanted anticholinergic effects (e.g., dry mouth, tachycardia, blurred vision, constipation) of the tricyclics. Although tolerance for some therapeutic effects, as in the case of hyperactivity, can be a real clinical problem, their antidepressant action remains present for long periods of time. There are, however, some reports of antidepressant tolerance with long-term MAO inhibitor therapy.

The drug withdrawal reactions of some patients (chills, muscle aches, vomiting, malaise, sweating, nasal stuffiness) indicate physical dependence. The types of withdrawal symptoms that are manifest suggest a cholinergic rebound effect. To prevent this reaction, gradual dosage reduction over a week or more is recommended when withdrawing medication.

Efficacy

The primary indications for antidepressant drug therapy are for the treatment of mood and anxiety disorders. In the pediatric age range, additional applications are in the management of hyperactivity, enuresis, and separation anxiety. In reviewing the literature on these diverse disorders, one is struck by the relatively high rate of placebo response and of symptom relapse subsequent to drug withdrawal. Although therapy is clearly effective for specific patients, many receive only mild to moderate benefit. Some cases of drug failure can be attributed to inadequate blood levels or noncompliance.

Anxiety Disorders. The antidepressants are used clinically in the management of several anxiety disorders, most notably panic disorder, obsessive compulsive disorder, and separation anxiety disorder. Of these, panic disorder is the most common in people seeking psychiatric treatment. The essential feature of this disorder is recurrent attacks of intense fear, discomfort, or feeling of impending doom, which usually last for several minutes. Obsessive compulsive disorder, the most treatment resistant of these conditions, is characterized by obsessions or compulsions that are severe enough to disrupt one's ability to function normally. In children, symptoms commonly take the form of repetitive thoughts of violence, contamination, or doubt and ritualistic actions involving handwashing, counting, checking, or touching (Flament et al., 1985). Separation anxiety disorder typically has an onset in early or middle childhood and is evidenced by excessive anxiety when separated from people to whom the child is attached. Because the diagnostic features of the anxiety disorders are presented in chapter 5, this discussion focuses on pharmacological considerations.

Panic disorder. Recurrent, spontaneous sudden episodes of fear, apprehension, or feelings of impending doom are referred to as panic disorder. Panic attack symptoms include difficulty breathing, *palpita-*

tions (heart beating hard and/or fast), chest pain, choking, dizziness, feelings of unreality, numbness in limbs, sweating, and faintness. There is often a feeling that one may die, go crazy, or lose control. A number of well-controlled studies have shown that imipramine and other tricyclics are effective for suppressing panic attacks in adults (Klein, 1981; Klein & Fink, 1962). Unfortunately, in typical treatment settings many patients stop taking tricyclic medication because they are unable (or unwilling) to tolerate the side effects (Noyes, Garvey, Cook & Samuelson, 1989). Two of the more troublesome are overstimulation (feeling keyed-up, jittery, and irritable) and weight gain. Because the disorder is rare in children and young adolescents, evidence supporting the drugs' efficacy in the pediatric age range is limited primarily to case reports.

The MAO inhibitors are useful for the treatment of panic attacks and may even be superior to tricyclics (Sheehan, Ballenger & Jacobsen, 1980). However, concerns about safety prevent their general acceptance as the drug of first choice.

Separation anxiety disorder. One common symptomatic manifestation of separation anxiety disorder is school refusal, and Gittelman-Klein and Klein (1971; Gittelman-Klein, 1975) showed that imipramine was superior to placebo in facilitating school attendance. Treatment with medication resulted in a considerable reduction in depression, severity of phobia, maternal dependence, physical complaints, and fear of going to school.

The average dose of imipramine for separation anxiety is 75 to 100 mg per day with a maximal upper limit of 200 mg per day. Although behavioral improvement may be evident immediately after the onset of treatment, it is more characteristically manifested sometime within the first 2 weeks. Unfortunately, many children who have a complete remission of symptoms with imipramine therapy later suffer relapses. Medication is often given before bedtime to avoid side effects (e.g., drowsiness, dry mouth). Total duration of treatment, including a gradual withdrawal period, lasts about 3 months. To be truly effective, treatment must include behavioral intervention strategies (which should be considered before a trial of medication) as well as the cooperation of the school, family, and child.

Obsessive compulsive disorder. There is evidence that at least some individuals with obsessive compulsive disorder have a chronic neurobiologic disturbance, often with a waxing and waning of symptomatology during their entire life cycle. Obsessive compulsive symptoms may also occur at some time during the course of schizophrenic, manic, or depressive illness and remit with appropriate treatment of the primary disorder. Obsessions are recurrent ideas, thoughts, images, or internal impulses that incessantly come to the level of consciousness and seem senseless or even distasteful to the person. Obsessions can be extremely varied and range from simple (e.g., an impulse to count numbers in one's head, to repeat words or phrases) to more complex mental activities. They may be related to fears of harm, infestation, or loss of self-control. Commonly, these obsessional thoughts are associated with ritualistic physical acts, such as repetitive washing, arrangement of objects, or movements of the body, which are collectively referred to as *compulsions*.

Recent studies have shown that the tricyclic antidepressant clomipramine (Anafranil), which was recently approved for use in the United States, is effective for the treatment of obsessive compulsive disorder in children, adolescents, and adults (reviewed by Elkins, Rapoport & Lipsky, 1980; Flament et al., 1985). Unfortunately, most drug responders do not recover fully, and there is typically a relapse in symptoms after drug withdrawal. Patients with compulsions respond better than those with obsessions only. Doses for children and adolescents range from 100 to 200 mg per day, and untoward reactions include tremor, dry mouth, dizziness, constipation, acute dyskinesia, and rarely tonic-clonic seizures.

Depression. A *major depressive episode* is characterized by either a depressed mood or a loss of interest or pleasure in all, or almost all, activities for at least 2 weeks in combination with at least four of the following associated symptoms: (a) significant weight loss or weight gain when not dieting or a decrease or increase in appetite, (b) difficulty sleeping or excessive sleep, (c) psychomotor agitation or retardation, (d) fatigue or loss of energy, (e) feelings of worthlessness or excessive or inappropriate guilt, (f) diminished ability to think or indecisiveness, and (g) recurrent thoughts of death or suicide (American Psychiatric Association, 1987). All symptoms pertain to a change from a previous level of functioning. Exclusion criteria include (a) the existence of organic factors that initiated or maintain the disturbance, (b) a normal reaction to the death of a loved one, (c) delusions or hallucinations for a period of at least 2 weeks in the absence of mood symptoms, and (d) psychosis. Commonly associated symptoms are anxiety, irritability, concerns about physical health, panic attacks, and phobias. Some patients experience hallucinations or delusions, the content of which reflects their mood. The average age of onset of a major depressive episode is the late 20s, but it may begin at any age. The onset may be gradual or sudden, and the typical duration is 6 months or longer if left untreated. The episode is usually followed by a complete remission of symptoms, but for some patients certain symptoms may persist for as long as 2 years. During the course of the episode, social and occupational (school) functioning is impaired to some degree.

A diagnosis of *major depression* is made for patients who experience one or more major depressive episodes and who have no history of manic or hypomanic episodes. Approximately 50% of patients who develop major depression experience additional episodes of depression. Those at greatest risk are patients with major depression superimposed on dysthymia (sometimes called *double depression*). The percentage of adults who meet the criteria for major depression at a specific point in time (point prevalence) is approximately 5% to 10% for females and 2% to 3% for males.

When depressive symptoms exist for at least 2 years (1 year for children and adolescents) without relief for more than 2 months, the patient is said to have *dysthymia*. It is different from major depression primarily on the basis of severity (dysthymia is usually characterized as mild), chronicity, and absence of discrete episodes of depression.

The evidence supporting the efficacy of antidepressants for the treatment of major depression in adults is compelling but not dramatic (Morris & Beck, 1974). Marked symptom suppression occurs in 65% to 85% of patients treated with tryicyclics, but 20% to 40% also improve with placebo (Baldessarini, 1989). The newer antidepressants have not been found to be more effective than the older tricyclics, but some patients who receive only marginal relief with the latter respond to the newer products (Cole, 1988). The most favorable response to tricyclics is achieved in patients whose symptoms are more severe and who exhibit vegetative (sleeping, eating) disturbances. The tricyclics and MAO inhibitors are equally effective, but the greater risk of toxicity for the latter explains their much more limited application. The onset of therapeutic action is slow for both classes of drugs, and a trial of an adequate dose requires approximately 1 month. However, when dosage is increased rapidly, therapeutic effects may be evident within a week. Blood level determinations are valuable for establishing whether the patient is in the therapeutic range and determining whether drug failure at high doses is due to subtherapeutic level of medication in the blood or, most importantly, whether side effects are the result of an unexpectedly high level of drug in the blood (Preskorn, 1989). Treatment is usually initiated with 50 mg per day of imipramine (or its equivalent), which is increased rapidly to 150 mg per day or more. Severely depressed hospitalized patients may require as much as 300 mg per day.

In selecting an antidepressant for a depressed patient, there is little to differentiate these drugs on the basis of efficacy. However, consideration of side effects can help in drug selection. When sedation is desirable at the onset of treatment, amitriptyline, doxepin, or trazo-done should be considered. When anticholinergic side effects are to be avoided, desipramine, trazodone, or fluoxetine are preferred (see Table 7.2).

Treatment is maintained for 3 to 6 months after full recovery because mood disorders have a high risk of recurrence. To avoid drug with-drawal reactions, dosage should be gradually reduced when treatment is terminated. Some clinicians employ a protracted dosage reduction schedule (over several months) based upon clinical response. Tricyclic therapy can be maintained for several years if necessary, either to ame-liorate symptoms or as a prophylaxis for recurring episodes.

Occasionally, patients predisposed to bipolar disorder "switch" to mania or even a *rapid cycling process* (continuous bouts of mania and depression; Wehr & Goodwin, 1979, 1987) during the course of treat-ment with an antidepressant (Strober & Carlson, 1982; Van Scheyen & Van Kamman, 1979). This is an indication to withdraw the antidepres-sant medication and use an antimanic drug. At the present time there is some controversy as to whether the switch is due to the pharmaco-logic properties of the antidepressant drug or is purely a part of the illness process (Lewis & Winokur, 1982). The risk of switching to mania following antidepressant drug therapy is low (3%) in patients who experience recurring episodes of depression (Kupfer, Carpenter & Frank, 1988).

In children. A great deal of interest has been generated over the ex-istence of depression in prepubertal children, and most of the research on this disorder has appeared within the last decade. Once considered a very rare condition, more recent surveys show that the prevalence of major depressive disorder in prepubertal children in the United States is approximately 1.8% (Kashani & Simonds, 1979). Many of the chil-dren who fit the criteria for depression are not taken for psychological or psychiatric help, and few are currently treated with medication (Ko-vacs, Feinberg, Crouse-Novak, Paulauskas & Finkelstein, 1984). Chil-dren with major depressive disorder are unlikely to recover within the first 3 months of the depressive episode, but remission generally oc-curs in 6 to 18 months. If the child does not recover by that time, the illness is likely to be protracted. The earlier the age of onset of the disorder, the longer the recovery period.

There are several reports (uncontrolled or case studies) on the use of tricyclic antidepressants for the treatment of major depressive dis-order in children, and some experts (e.g., Puig-Antich, 1982) have stated that significant clinical improvement can be realized at higher thera-peutic doses. However, a well-controlled study of a fairly large sample of depressed prepubertal children failed to show that imipramine was superior to placebo in diminishing depressive symptoms (Puig-Antich et al., 1987). Some reviewers of the literature on pharmacotherapy for prepubertal depressed children also question the existence of a clinically significant therapeutic response to medication in many cases (e.g., Ambrosini, 1987). Therefore, caution is warranted when prescribing drug therapy for this disorder, and appropriate child- and family-oriented psychological interventions are the treatments of choice.

Children who meet the diagnostic criteria for major depressive disorder may also experience other psychiatric problems as well. Many have conduct disorders (Carlson & Cantwell, 1980; Puig-Antich, 1982) or exhibit antisocial behavior (Geller, Chestnut, Miller, Price & Yates, 1985), anxiety disorder (Kovacs et al., 1984), separation anxiety (Geller et al., 1985), school phobia (Kolvin et al., 1984), or psychotic symptoms such as hallucinations or delusions (Freeman et al., 1985). For these children, the total treatment plan is complicated by the presence of multiple target behaviors, some of which may become the reason for pharmacotherapy.

In adolescents. The commonest pharmacological treatment of adolescent depression is also tricyclic medication, particularly imipramine, amitriptyline, and desipramine. In adolescents, the therapeutic dose of these drugs ranges up to 5 mg/kg per day, whereas the average dose of nortriptyline is 1 to 2 mg/kg per day (Ryan & Puig-Antich, 1987). Imipramine can be safely administered as a single dose at night, particularly once a steady state has been achieved (Ryan et al., 1987). The best indicators that a depressed adolescent will respond to antidepressant medication are the presence of so-called vegetative (biological) symptoms such as sleep disturbance, change in eating patterns, and lack of drive, particularly if there is also a family history of depression.

The findings from controlled studies of tricyclic drug treatment in depressed adolescents have not been particularly compelling. Kramer and Feiguine (1981) showed no advantage for amitriptyline 200 mg per day over placebo in 10 adolescent inpatients with major depression. Ryan et al. (1986) found that less than half of their sample of 34 depressed adolescents had a complete recovery within 4 weeks of a final-weight adjusted dose of imipramine (mean = 234 mg per day), but all had at least a partial response. No relationship was found between plasma level and clinical response. Because the tricyclics are among the more commonly used drugs for attempted suicide in this age group (Fazen, Lovejoy & Crone, 1986), medication should be administered and safely stored by the parent. Adolescents who do not respond favorably to an adequate trial of tricyclic medication may show improvement with the addition of lithium carbonate to the treatment regimen. Research on this practice is limited, but nevertheless encouraging (Ryan, Meyer, Dachille, Mazzie & Puig-Antich, 1988a).

The medical literature on the use of MAO inhibitors for depressed children and adolescents consists largely of anecdotal reports or poorly controlled studies. The indications for their use in adolescents are limited to intractable depression (Ryan et al., 1988b) and severe emotional disorders.

It is important to realize that depressive symptoms are often observed in association with environmental stress (e.g., death of a loved one), drug and alcohol abuse, physical illness, and other psychiatric disorders. Focusing treatment on the depressive symptoms instead of the youth's problems may be ineffective or even detrimental.

In the elderly. Depressive syndromes are relatively common in the elderly, particularly those who are hospitalized for medical illnesses. Diagnosis is often complicated by the presence of chronic physical illnesses, memory impairment, and mild to moderate dementia, and the patient's focus on physical rather than affective complaints. The findings from drug studies with elderly patients (reviewed by Gerson, Plotkin & Jarvik, 1988) indicate that doxepin, nortriptyline, and desipramine can be used effectively with this population. Antidepressants that produce moderate to high rates of anticholinergic side effects (e.g., imipramine, amitriptyline) are to be avoided. For example, imipramine-induced orthostatic hypotension can cause the patient to fall, possibly causing a hip fracture. Perhaps the best dosage selection and titration guideline is to start low and go slow (Small, 1989). Alternative agents should be considered when low to moderate doses are ineffective.

Medical treatment for serious mood disorders is recommended for all age groups. Although these disorders are self-limiting, appropriate medical management significantly reduces the length and severity of disturbance and the risk of harm either through self-neglect or suicide. Management consists of both therapy for the acute illness and long-term treatment for prevention of recurrence.

Enuresis. In an excellent review of the literature, Blackwell and Currah (1973) stated that the tricyclic antidepressants are the only drugs that have consistently proved to be more effective than placebo for the treatment of *nocturnal enuresis* (bed wetting). Several different tricyclics have been found to be effective, but imipramine is the most commonly used for this disorder. It was first reported as a treatment for enuresis by MacLean in 1960 and 13 years later was approved by the FDA for use with this disorder.

When imipramine works, the response is immediate, usually during the first week of treatment. A complete cure (total remission of symptoms), however, is reported for less than half of the children on medication. It should be noted that if a less stringent criterion is used (e.g., 50% fewer wet nights), the "success" rate is much higher. Unfortunately, "relapse tends to occur immediately following withdrawal after short periods of treatment, and long-term followup studies suggest that total remission (no wet nights) occurs in only a minority of patients" (Blackwell & Currah, 1973, p. 253).

The total daily dose of imipramine commonly reported in the literature is 25 to 50 mg given in one oral dose at bedtime. For children over 12 years of age, the dose may be increased to 75 mg if the smaller amount is unsuccessful. The FDA recommends that the dose of imipramine not exceed 2.5 mg/kg per day because there is a risk of severe side effects at higher doses (Robinson & Barker, 1976).

Day wetting is referred to as *diurnal enuresis*. This condition is more common in females and is often associated with behavior problems at home and at school (Meadow & Berg, 1982). It is a difficult disorder to treat successfully (i.e., no relapses). In one study that examined the utility of two different doses of imipramine (25 mg and 50 mg administered in the morning) for diurnal enuresis, Meadow and Berg (1982) found that medication was not more effective than placebo.

The treatment of first choice for nocturnal enuresis is the buzzer-pad procedure, which may or may not be incorporated into a more elaborate behavior therapy program (Schaffer, 1985). Medication should be considered only when proven behavioral interventions have failed or are not practical or when special circumstances warrant, such as vacations or highly stressful home settings. Studies comparing psychological and pharmacological treatments for enuresis have resulted in mixed findings. For example, Kolvin et al. (1972) examined the relative efficacy of imipramine, conditioning, and placebo. Children in the study were separated into three groups, each receiving one of the aforementioned treatments. Therapy for each group lasted 2 months, with the results being evaluated 2 months later. Treatment was considered successful if there was an 80% decrease in wet nights. Using this criterion, 42% of the placebo group, 30% of the medication group, and 50% of the buzzer-pad group were considered improved. Conversely, Wagner, Johnson, Walker, Carter, and Wittner (1982) found tricyclic antidepressants to be superior to the buzzer-pad in a short-term study.

Hyperactivity (Attention-deficit Hyperactivity Disorder). Imipramine was once considered the drug of second choice for the treatment of hyperactivity on the basis of findings from several studies (e.g., Rapoport, Quinn, Bradbard, Riddle & Brooks 1974; Werry, Aman & Diamond, 1980). Unfortunately, many children appear to develop a tolerance for the therapeutic response (Quinn & Rapoport, 1975). There are some data to suggest that hyperactive children who (a) are more difficult to manage in the evening hours, (b) have mood disturbance symptoms, or (c) are highly anxious may be more responsive to imipramine than stimulant drugs (Pliszka, 1987). The total daily dose of imipramine ranges from 50 to 200 mg, usually divided into three doses of 50 mg or 75 mg per day. Some recent studies also indicate that desipramine is an effective treatment for some hyperactive children (Biederman, Baldessarini, Wright, Knee & Harmatz, 1989).

Untoward Effects

Tricyclic antidepressants often produce side effects that are troublesome but rarely dangerous. Their anticholinergic effects include dry mouth, sour or metallic taste in the mouth, nausea, constipation, dizziness, increased heart rate, blurred vision, and rarely an inability to pass urine (urinary retention). Other complaints include weakness, fatigue, and excessive sweating. Older patients are more likely to report dizziness, orthostatic hypotension, constipation, urinary retention, swelling, and muscle tremors. The latter can be treated with small doses of propranolol. Confusion or delirium is a common reaction in adult patients, particularly those over the age of 50. Treatment with neuroleptics can exacerbate these confusional states. The best course of action is to withdraw the antidepressant.

Another major complication of the tricyclics is their effect on nerve conduction within the heart muscle. Therapeutic levels of the tricyclics can produce changes in heart function that register on EKG records, and susceptible individuals may develop unusual heart rhythms or a "racing" of the heart (tachycardia). During treatment it is therefore imperative for the physician to assess heart function thoroughly. It is recommended that an EKG be obtained prior to the onset of treatment to determine if there is a preexisting heart disorder and after each increase in dosage (Ryan & Puig-Antich, 1987). The effect on the heart is one of the main reasons why these drugs can be very lethal in overdose (accidental or not), an important consideration when treating children or adolescents, particularly those with suicidal ideas. The risk to the heart is also the reason why a single nighttime dose may be ill advised in preadolescent children, because they are more likely to develop toxic blood levels than adolescents.

The effects of tricyclic medication on cognitive and academic performance have not been studied extensively, but most reports with children are encouraging. The tricyclics have some actions that are similar to the stimulants, which probably account for their beneficial effect on some hyperactive children such as increasing attention span and decreasing impulsivity (Rapoport et al., 1974; Yepes, Balka, Winsberg & Bialer, 1977). There is also evidence that long-term tricyclic treatment does not cause deterioration in academic performance (Quinn & Rapoport, 1975).

Additional side effects that are rare but nevertheless potentially serious are extrapyramidal syndromes, including tardive dyskinesia (Yassa, Camille & Belzile, 1987) and akathisia (Zubenko, Cohen & Lipinski, 1987), glaucoma, and tonic-clonic seizures, particularly in children (Brown, Winsberg, Bialer & Press, 1973). The effect on seizure threshold is greatest for maprotiline in doses above 250 mg (Rotblatt, 1982) and least for desipramine.

With regard to the atypical antidepressants, trazodone has less anticholinergic activity and subsequently fewer autonomic nervous system side effects. However, trazodone can cause *priapism* (persistent penile erection) and permanent impotence (Lansky & Selzer, 1984). Of all the antidepressants discussed in this chapter, the risk of drug-induced seizures is greatest for buproprion. Two of the more common side effects of fluoxetine are gastrointestinal distress and anxiety.

Some side effects of the MAO inhibitors are similar to those of the tricyclics and include dizziness, vertigo, headache, inhibition of ejaculation, urinary retention, weakness, fatigue, dry mouth, orthostatic hypotension, blurred vision, skin rashes, and constipation. Liver toxicity is rare but potentially serious. CNS reactions include tremor, insomnia, excessive sweating, agitation, *hypomania* (mild degree of mania), and rarely hallucinations and confusion. The main concern with these drugs is the potential for life-threatening reactions when treated individuals eat food containing tyramine or are given a number of different medications (see Drug Interactions). The combination of MAO inhibitors and these substances can produce a rapid rise in blood pressure. It is therefore important that the patient who is administered a MAO inhibitor (a) takes medication in the prescribed manner, (b) follows all dietary restrictions, and (c) avoids illicit drugs, particularly cocaine, amphetamine, and methamphetamine (speed).

Drug Interactions

The tricyclic antidepressants interact with a number of other commonly used drugs and substances. Because the tricyclics are highly bound to plasma proteins, other highly bound drugs that compete for these binding sites can displace the former, resulting in elevated levels of unbound tricyclic drug molecules in the blood. Some examples of drugs that can affect the tricyclics in this manner are aspirin, aminophyllin (an antiasthmatic), phenothiazines (see chapter 4), phenylbutazone (an analgesic), phenytoin (see chapter 8), and scopolamine (for motion sickness). Blood levels of tricyclic medication also rise when biotransformation is inhibited by drugs such as methylphenidate (see chapter 6), neuroleptics (see chapter 4), and oral contraceptives. Tricyclic blood levels may drop when given in combination with drugs that induce liver enzymes that metabolize the tricyclics. Examples of such inducers are barbiturates (chapter 5) and cigarette smoking.

Tricyclics can potentiate the effects of alcohol, norepinephrine, and amphetamine. Because tricyclics have anticholinergic actions, side effects must be carefully monitored when they are administered in combination with other anticholinergic medications such as antiparkinsonian agents and neuroleptics (see chapter 4). Tricyclics can also block the effect of guanethidine (an antihypertensive agent). The concurrent administration of a tricyclic and a MAO inhibitor can produce a rare but severe reaction marked by fever, convulsions, and coma.

Because the MAO inhibitors interfere with various bodily enzymes, they can prolong and intensify the effects of other drugs such as neurotransmitter precursors (e.g., levodopa), sympathomimetic amines (e.g., amphetamine, tyramine), CNS depressants (anesthetics, sedatives, antihistamines, alcohol, potent analgesics), anticholinergic agents, and antidepressants (especially imipramine and amitriptyline). The most serious toxic reaction as a result of a drug interaction is hypertensive crisis, which results from eating foods that contain relatively large amounts of the amino acid tyramine. Such foods include aged cheeses, beer, wine, yeast extract, liver, citrus fruits, yogurt, broad bean pods, and cream. Excessive amounts of caffeine and chocolate can also cause hypertensive reactions. The hypertensive crisis occurs because insufficient amounts of MAO are available in the liver and other organs to metabolize tyramine and similar substances, which then stimulate the release of neurotransmitters that cause heart rate and blood pressure to increase dramatically. Headache and fever are commonly associated symptoms.

LITHIUM SALTS

Lithium salts (usually lithium carbonate) were first used in medicine in the 1800s as a treatment for gout. In the 1940s lithium chloride became a much-touted salt substitute for cardiac and other patients, but its popularity abruptly ceased when reports of toxicity and death began to appear. During this time period in Australia, Cade was experimenting with lithium salts in guinea pigs and noted that it made them lethargic, which prompted him to initiate clinical trials with agitated or manic psychiatric patients. He subsequently reported a specific effect for mania (Cade, 1949). Lithium chloride's prior track record of toxicity, however, diminished enthusiasm for the new treatment, and not until 1970 was it recognized by the FDA as a treatment for mania in the United States (Gattozzi, 1970).

Pharmacology

Lithium ions are readily absorbed from the gastrointestinal tract, and peak blood concentrations are reached 2 to 4 hours after a single oral dose (Amdisen, 1969; Lydiard & Gelenberg, 1982). Lithium ions are not bound to plasma proteins. Passage through the blood–brain barrier is slow. Lithium ions are not metabolized in any way and are excreted almost entirely by the kidneys. Small amounts appear in feces, sweat, and breast milk; and breast-feeding infants is contraindicated during active stages of lithium treatment.

Mechanism of Action

The mechanism of action for lithium's antimanic effect is unknown. Numerous theories have been formulated, which have focused on (a) the distribution of sodium, calcium, and magnesium ions, (b) the inhibition of norepinephrine and dopamine activity through various mechanisms, and (c) the alteration of cellular transport mechanisms, which reduces neuronal responsivity to neurotransmitters.

Dose and Schedule

Lithium is the only drug in current use in psychiatry for which blood levels correlate highly with clinical response. Blood levels between approximately 1.0 and 1.5 mEq/L are considered optimal for acute manic episodes. (The term mEq/L refers to milliequivalents, which is a measure of the number of lithium ions in a liter of blood.) Blood levels above 1.5 mEq/L generally result in lithium toxicity, whereas levels below 0.9 mEq/L are typically ineffective. In milligrams the oral dose is generally in the range of 900 to 1,500 mg per day for outpatients and 1,200 to 2,400 mg per day for inpatients. Blood levels between 0.75 and 1.0 mEq/L are usually satisfactory for long-term prophylaxis.

When treatment is initiated, dosage is increased every 3 to 4 days. Approximately 12 hours after each dosage increment, a blood sample is taken for laboratory analysis. This is sometimes referred to as the 12-hour standardized lithium concentration (12 hst SLi). When the optimal dose is reached, it is generally recommended that a drug blood analysis be conducted once a month. It takes approximately 5 days for lithium ions to reach a steady state in the blood. Therapeutic response for manic episodes usually develops in 6 to 10 days after optimal blood level is reached. For some patients, full protection against depressive relapses does not develop until after weeks or months of continuous treatment.

Although the half-life of lithium is 20 to 24 hours, it is generally administered in divided doses to minimize the possibility of adverse reactions. Lithium carbonate is available in the United States as 300-mg tablets and capsules and slow-release formulations (typically administered twice daily) and as a liquid (lithium citrate). Lithium is never administered parenterally.

Because the dosage adjustment phase of lithium treatment is somewhat protracted (which delays the onset of the therapeutic response), requires repeated venipunctures, and is not currently approved by the Food and Drug Administration for children under 12 years of age, its application for prepubertal disorders has been limited but is nevertheless becoming more widely accepted (reviewed by Campbell et al., 1984a). Weller, Weller, and Fristad (1986) have developed a dosing procedure for children that enables the clinician to achieve a therapeutic blood level in 5 days. The key to this procedure is to start treatment with a relatively large dose of medication, which is possible in children because they eliminate lithium from their bodies at a faster rate than adults. Monitoring of saliva level may eventually offer a feasible alternative to blood level analyses (see Weller et al., 1986), but some clinicians have found this not to be a suitable substitute (Perry, Campbell, Grega & Anderson, 1984).

Efficacy

The primary indication for lithium treatment is bipolar disorder (mania, manic-depressive illness). However, it is also effective for the treatment of severe recurrent depression (and is sometimes used as an alternative for the tricyclics) and may be used in combination with an antidepressant for the treatment of major depressive episode. There is also considerable interest in its application for episodic childhood behavioral disturbances and conduct disorder (aggression).

Aggression. There is a growing number of reports on the efficacy of lithium treatment for aggressive behavior. Campbell et al. (1984b), for example, conducted a thorough and well-controlled investigation into the effects of haloperidol and lithium on hospitalized conduct-disordered, undersocialized, aggressive children between 5 and 13 years old. The optimal dose of lithium was 500 to 2,000 mg per day (or serum levels of 0.32 to 1.51 mEq/L). Both haloperidol and lithium were highly effective in reducing aggressive behavior. Qualitatively, haloperidol rendered the children more manageable, whereas lithium reduced the explosive nature of their aggressive behavior, which enabled other positive changes to take place. Subjectively, the children receiving haloperidol felt "slowed down," and the youngsters getting lithium thought that medication "helped to control" themselves. It appeared that the optimal dose of haloperidol interfered with daily functioning more than lithium.

Lithium has shown some effectiveness as an antiaggression agent for some mentally retarded people (reviewed by Gadow & Poling, 1988), epileptic patients, and neurologically normal male delinquents (reviewed by Sheard, 1978). Among the latter group, certain characteristics seem to be associated with effectiveness of lithium treatment: mood lability (rapid changes between euphoria and depression), irritability, hostility, restlessness, impulsivity, distractibility, *pressured speech* (excessive, rapid talking), and a loud and provocative manner. Other researchers have described a similar personality profile among adolescent females, which they have called the emotionally unstable character disorder (Rifkin, Quitkin, Carillo, Blumberg & Klein, 1972). This disorder is also purported to show a response to lithium therapy. The doses of lithium recommended in these studies are the same as those used to control mania.

Bipolar Illness. A *manic episode* is characterized by "a distinct period of abnormally and persistently elevated, expansive, or irritable mood" associated with three of the following: inflated self-esteem or grandiosity, decreased need for sleep, talkativeness, flight of ideas or racing thoughts, distractibility, increased level of activity, and excessive involvement in pleasurable activities that ultimately have negative consequences (American Psychiatric Association, 1987). Exclusion criteria are (a) delusions or hallucinations in the absence of mood symptoms, (b) psychosis, and (c) clearly identifiable organic basis for the disturbances. The average age at onset is the early 20s. Manic episodes are sometimes brief (a few days), but they may last for months. If the mood disturbance is not severe enough to impair social or occupational (school) function, it is referred to as a hypomanic episode. Patients who experience one or more manic episodes, usually in conjunction with one or more depressive episodes, are said to have *bipolar disorder*. Usually the first episode that requires hospitalization is manic, and the episodes of mania and depression occur more frequently than in major depression.

When patients experience two or more complete cycles of mania followed immediately by depression (or vice versa) within a single year, they are said to have a *rapid cycling* disorder. Approximately 0.5% to 1% of the adult population have had bipolar disorder, and it is equally prevalent in males and females. Onset is usually during adolescence or early adulthood.

An episode of mania is a serious medical problem and typically requires hospitalization. Treatment is generally initiated with a neuroleptic in order to render the patient more manageable. After symptoms stabilize and the patient becomes more compliant, treatment with lithium can be initiated. Its most important therapeutic role is the prevention of recurring episodes of both mania and depression. Because the tricyclics can provoke a switch to mania, it is often recommended to treat a bipolar patient who is experiencing an acute depressive episode with a combination of an antidepressant and lithium. Lithium is less effective in preventing mood swings in patients with rapid cycling bipolar disorder, but it can decrease the duration of each individual mood swing and the overall severity of the manic episode (Dunner, Vijayalasky & Fieve, 1977).

The duration of maintenance therapy for the prevention of manic and depressive episodes depends in part upon the severity of the disorder, the frequency of recurrence, and patient compliance, which may be influenced by side effects. Two of the more disturbing adverse reactions for patients receiving maintenance lithium treatment are cognitive effects (e.g., poor concentration, memory problems, mental confusion, mental slowness) and weight gain (Gitlin, Cochran & Jamison, 1989).

In children and adolescents. Bipolar disorder is considered to be a rare condition in prepubertal children, and there is no consensus of opinion about its diagnostic features. It has been described by DeLong (1978) as a condition characterized by "cyclic or periodic hostile aggressiveness; extremes of mood including manic excitement, depression, and angry irritability; distractibility; neurovegetative disorders (hyperdipsia, hyperphagia, encopresis, salt or sugar craving, excess sweating); and a family history of affective disorder" (DeLong & Aldershof, 1987, p. 389). Children exhibiting such symptoms may be responsive to treatment with lithium, implying but not confirming a continuity with adult bipolar disorder.

Lithium is effective in treating mania in adolescents (Carlson, 1983, 1986) but in the initial phase of the illness, it is commonly given in combination with a neuroleptic because the latter helps the adolescent calm down. Long-term pharmacotherapy with lithium is considered appropriate when (a) there is clear evidence of often-recurring episodes of mood disorder and (b) the manic episodes are disruptive enough to warrant the risks of such treatment. Adolescents reportedly tolerate larger doses of lithium than adults because they tend to excrete lithium through their kidneys more rapidly than older people.

Schizophrenia. Research has not established the efficacy of lithium as a general treatment for chronic schizophrenia. However, some patients diagnosed as being schizophrenic, primarily those with a family history of affective disorder, active affective symptoms, or previous affective episodes, may respond favorably to lithium (Atre-Vaidya & Taylor, 1989).

Untoward Reactions

The side effects of lithium include nausea, headache, *fine tremor* (slight trembling or shaking, usually of the hands), sleepiness, thirst, *polyuria* (excessive need to urinate), and diarrhea. Signs of acute intoxication are vomiting, diarrhea, shaking, mental confusion, slurred speech, dizziness, seizures, and coma. Other toxic effects are cardiac arrhythmias and hypotension. Adequate salt and fluid intake is required to prevent toxic levels of lithium from developing. This is particularly important during warm weather, which may lead to fluid loss from sweating. Concerns about long-term adverse reactions include potentially irreversible effects on the kidney, thyroid, and possibly bone (Birch, 1980). None of these problems has proven to be common, and they can be easily monitored by regular testing of chemical and hormonal levels in the blood. Because there is a risk of birth defects with lithium treatment (Weinstein, 1980), it should be used with caution for women who may become pregnant.

The effects of lithium on cognitive function are unclear. In normal volunteers, lithium can induce apathy, impair word learning, and reduce performance on visual-motor tasks, but studies of patients on long-term lithium therapy have found no gross impairment on standardized intelligence test performance (Judd, Squire, Butters, Salmon & Paller, 1987). It seems reasonable to conclude that for patients with severe recurrent mood disorder, neither side effects nor fear of cognitive deterioration are sufficient reasons not to use lithium in appropriate cases.

Drug Interactions

There are no firm contraindications regarding the use of lithium in combination with other psychotropic drugs. There are, nevertheless, reports of CNS toxicity when given in combination with haloperidol, but many patients appear not to be affected adversely (see Tupin & Schuller, 1978). The combination of lithium and a tricyclic can result in an extremely uncomfortable situation when the tricyclic induces urinary retention and lithium causes diuresis. Lithium decreases the euphoric effect of cocaine and other stimulants. Diuretics can alter lithium blood levels.

CONCLUDING COMMENT

Although they are used primarily to treat mood disorders, the antidepressant and antimanic drugs have a wide and expanding range of clinical applications. Unfortunately, these medications do not benefit all patients, and they are capable of producing a variety of untoward reactions. For these reasons, careful monitoring of individuals treated with them is of critical importance.

Chapter 8
Antiepileptic Drugs

Although antiepileptic drugs typically are used to manage seizures, they are included in this book because (a) they are behaviorally active and (b) they are likely to be prescribed in combination with psychotropic agents, especially in mentally retarded people (Gadow & Poling, 1988). Moreover, certain antiepileptic drugs, including carbamazepine, phenytoin, and valproic acid, occasionally are prescribed to treat behavior disorders. Carbamazepine in particular shows promise as a psychotropic medication. As the use of antiepileptic drugs in managing behavior disorders is not yet well established, the present chapter will focus on these medications as employed to control epileptic seizures.

EPILEPSY AND THE CLASSIFICATION OF SEIZURES

As stated by Rall and Schleifer (1985),

> The term epilepsies is a collective designation of a group of chronic CNS disorders having in common the occurrence of sudden and transitory episode (seizures) of abnormal phenomena of motor (convulsions), sensory, autonomic, or psychic origin. The seizures are nearly always correlated with abnormal and excessive EEG discharges. (p. 446)

The term *primary* or *idiopathic* epilepsy is applied to those cases where no cause can be found; *secondary* or *symptomatic* epilepsy designates cases where known causal factors are present. Among the factors known to cause epilepsy are traumatic brain injury, oxygen and nutritional deficiencies, infections of the central nervous system, toxic conditions (e.g., drug overdoses), cerebrovascular diseases, and brain tumors

(Howell, 1978). The majority of cases of epilepsy are of the primary type. Hauser (1978) estimates that the prevalence of all forms of epilepsy in the general population is 0.3% to 0.6%, but the Epilepsy Foundation of America (1975) cites a considerably higher prevalence rate of 2%. The prevalence is greater among mentally retarded individuals and increases with the degree of retardation. Epilepsy also is relatively common among autistic and brain-injured individuals.

Epilepsy takes several forms, which are differentiated on the basis of the type of seizures that occur. Seizures are classified according to clinical manifestations and characteristic EEG (electroencephalograph) patterns. There are a number of different schemes for classifying seizures, and the same seizure type may be assigned different names by different individuals. For example, what are now widely termed generalized tonic-clonic seizures were once commonly called grand mal seizures, and today's absence seizures were once termed petit mal seizures. Because the older terms are familiar to many individuals and continue to be employed, they will be used parenthetically in the present chapter. Detailed information concerning the classification of seizures is provided by the Commission on Classification and Terminology of the International League Against Epilepsy (1981). Table 8.1 summarizes the most salient characteristics of various seizure forms.

The most common type of seizure, the *tonic-clonic* (grand mal), consists of two phases. In the tonic phase, which appears first, the body becomes rigid, consciousness is lost, and breathing grows heavy and irregular. Drooling, skin pallor, and urinary incontinence may occur. This is followed by the clonic phase, which is characterized by acute muscular spasms, most readily observed in the muscles of the jaw and legs. The clonic phase is frequently followed by postconvulsive phenomena that include headache, sleep, disorientation, and fatigue. Tonic-clonic seizures sometimes are preceded by *auras*, which frequently take the form of a peculiar sensation (e.g., smell or taste) or a sense of impending doom.

Absence (petit mal) seizures are more difficult for an untrained observer to detect than tonic-clonic seizures. Absence seizures are characterized by short and sudden lapses of consciousness during which the individual often appears to be absently staring into space. Motor movements, including lip smacking, chewing, and eye blinking, are common. The eyes sometimes roll back, and clonic (jerking) movements of the eyebrows, eyelids, and head are observed in some patients. Absence seizures typically occur in children. The seizures are brief (less than 1 minute) in duration, but may occur in clusters (100 or more seizures per day is not unknown). Behavior typically is not dramatically altered following the occurrence of absence seizures.

Table 8.1. Classification of Epileptic Seizures

Seizure Type	Characteristics
Partial Seizures	
A. Simple partial seizures	Various manifestations, without impairment of consciousness, including convulsions confined to a single limb or muscle group *(Jacksonian motor epilepsy)*, specific and localized sensory disturbances *(Jacksonian sensory epilepsy)*, and other limited signs and symptoms depending upon the particular cortical area producing the abnormal discharge
B. Complex partial seizures	Attacks of confused behavior, with impairment of consciousness, with a wide variety of clinical manifestations, associated with bizarre generalized EEG activity during the seizure but with evidence of anterior temporal lobe focal abnormalities even in the interseizure period in many cases
C. Partial seizures secondarily generalized	
Generalized Seizures	
A.1. Absence seizures	Brief and abrupt loss of consciousness associated with high-voltage, bilaterally synchronous, 3-per-second spike-and-wave pattern in the EEG, usually with some symmetrical clonic motor activity varying from eyelid blinking to jerking of the entire body, sometimes with no motor activity
A.2. Atypical absence seizures	Attacks with slower onset and cessation than is usual for absence seizures, associated with a more heterogeneous EEG
B. Myoclonic seizures	Isolated clonic jerks associated with brief bursts of multiple spikes in the EEG
C. Clonic seizures	Rhythmic clonic contractions of all muscles, loss of consciousness, and marked autonomic manifestations
D. Tonic seizures	Opisthotonus [a backward arched position of the body in which the feet and head touch the floor], loss of consciousness, and marked autonomic manifestations
E. Tonic-clonic seizures	Major convulsions, usually a sequence of maximal tonic spasm of all body musculature followed by a synchronous clonic jerking and a prolonged depression of all central functions
F. Atonic seizures	Loss of postural tone, with sagging of the head or falling

Note: From "Drugs Effective in the Therapy of the Epilepsies," by T. W. Rall and L. S. Schleifer, 1990, in *The Pharmacological Basis of Therapeutics* (p. 437) by A. G. Gilman, T. W. Rall, A. S. Nies, and P. Taylor (Eds.). Elmsford, New York: Pergamon Press. Reproduced by permission.

Tonic-clonic and absence seizures are *generalized*. That is, the abnormal electrical activity associated with them occurs on both sides of the brain (i.e., bilaterally and symmetrically), and its origin is not localized in either cerebral hemisphere. In contrast to generalized seizures, *partial* (or focal) seizures begin in a circumscribed part of one cerebral hemisphere. *Simple partial seizures* (cortical focal seizures) involve localized motor or sensory disturbances and are not associated with loss of consciousness. *Complex partial seizures* (temporal lobe and psychomotor seizures) entail impaired consciousness and a wide range of motor and sensory responses, which frequently resemble those associated with absence seizures. Complex partial seizures are most common in older children or adults, have a duration of several minutes, and frequently are preceded by an aura.

Immediate temporal antecedents of seizures are not apparent in most cases of epilepsy, but specifiable environmental, physiological, and psychological changes do in some cases precede seizures (Rall & Schleifer, 1985). Among them are changes in blood glucose level, plasma pH, electrolyte compositions of extracellular fluid, and blood gas tensions. Fatigue, poor diet, hyperventilation, exposure to sudden sounds or lights flashing at particular frequencies, and emotional stress may precipitate seizures in some individuals.

Clinical symptoms and EEG records form the basis for diagnosing epilepsy and for differentiating seizure types. The EEG measures the amplitude and pattern of electrical (i.e., neuronal) activity at various parts of the brain. By comparing a patient's EEG recordings to control recordings, the neurological locus of seizure activity can be determined and accurate diagnosis accomplished. For example, the overt features of absence and complex partial seizures are often similar, but the EEG patterns associated with them are clearly different (Gibbs et al., 1982).

Although seizures are accompanied by unusual electrical activity in the brain, which is evident in abnormal EEG patterns, the converse is not necessarily true: In some individuals, EEG patterns are abnormal relative to controls, but there is no accompanying disruption of ongoing behaviors. Some authorities suggest that it is judicious to medicate on the basis of abnormal EEG recordings alone. For example, Gibbs et al. (1982) note that, "Not all EEG abnormalities correlate with symptoms of epilepsy but it is reasonable and prudent to treat EEG abnormalities on the basis of statistical probabilities for the expression of symptoms rather than waiting for the symptoms to be expressed" (p. 280). But, in view of the deleterious side effects associated with all antiepileptic medications (addressed later), a seemingly strong case can be made against administering such drugs to individuals who derive no obvious benefit from them.

Appropriate diagnosis of seizure type is crucial, for this determines the kind of medication that is likely to be useful. Although considerable gains have been made in the classification and diagnosis of seizure disorders, the appropriate interpretation of EEG records and clinical symptoms remains in some cases difficult. For example, Hooshmand (1978) has shown that commercial laboratories sometimes vary in their interpretation of the same EEG records, with some producing inaccurate interpretations. The possibility of inaccuracy in initial assessment, coupled with the realization that epilepsy is a dynamic disorder with features that can change over time, dictates that EEG records and clinical symptoms should be evaluated at regular intervals.

Extreme care must be taken not to confuse *pseudoepileptic seizures*, or *pseudoseizures*, with true seizures. Pseudoseizures superficially resemble true seizures, but are not accompanied by EEG alterations or altered consciousness. Pseudoseizures are most common in children with a history of epilepsy and apparently are maintained by their consequences, such as attention from adults (Goodyer, 1985). Medication should not be used to treat pseudoseizures, which are well controlled by behavioral interventions (Williams & Mostofsky, 1982). Unfortunately, it can be difficult to differentiate pseudoseizures from true epilepsy. According to Goodyer (1985), the former typically are accompanied by marked anxiety and hyperventilation, and no changes in behavior are observed when they end. These features should alert caregivers to the possibility of pseudoseizures. Procedures that allow the EEG to be recorded in the natural environment (see Stores, 1985) may be required for final diagnosis in some cases.

TREATMENT OF
SEIZURE DISORDERS

Except when prolonged (as in *status epilepticus*), seizures usually do not pose a direct and serious threat to a person's health. Seizures nonetheless require treatment for two important reasons. The first is that loss of consciousness for even a moment can be dangerous, even life-threatening, depending upon what the person is doing when the seizure occurs. The second is that the social consequences of public seizures are troublesome to most people with epilepsy.

Although other treatments, such as behavior modification, are sometimes used successfully, drugs provide the most effective and most often used means of controlling epilepsy. The success of pharmacotherapy is related to the type of seizure and the extent of associated neurological abnormalities.

Several different drugs are used to manage epilepsy (Table 8.2), although the majority of them are prescribed infrequently. Carbamazepine (Tegretol), phenytoin (Dilantin), valproic acid (Depakene), and phenobarbital (Luminal) are the antiepileptic drugs used most commonly and will be emphasized here.

Because many patients have more than one type of seizure, polypharmacy (the simultaneous prescription of two or more drugs) is common in the treatment of epilepsy. Multiple drug therapy also is sometimes employed when a single seizure type is evident. The aim here is to enhance seizure control or reduce side effects relative to single drug therapy. According to a National Epilepsy League survey (Pietsch, 1977), 71% of epileptic children receive more than one drug. Common among drug combinations are phenytoin and phenobarbital, phenytoin and primidone, and primidone and phenobarbital (Gadow & Kalachnik, 1981). Combinations involving three or more drugs also are sometimes prescribed, most often when seizures are difficult to control. Although polypharmacy is commonplace in the management of epilepsy, some researchers (e.g., Reynolds & Shorvon, 1981) have suggested that a single drug employed appropriately frequently can be substituted for drug combinations with no loss of seizure control or increase in side effects.

Detailed coverage of all the drugs and drug combinations employed in dealing with particular seizure types and of the strategies employed in their selection is beyond the scope of this chapter. Readers inter-

Table 8.2. Generic and (in parentheses) Trade Names of Antiepileptic Drugs. Many of These Drugs are Rarely Prescribed.

Barbiturates	**Benzodiazepines**
mephobarbital (Mebaral)	clonazepam (Klonopin)
metharbital (Gemonil)	clorazepate (Tranxene)
phenobarbital (Luminal)	diazepam (Valium)
primidone (Mysoline)[a]	**Succinimides**
Hydantoins	ethosuximide (Zarontin)
ethotoin (Peganone)	methsuximide (Celontin)
mephenytoin (Mesantoin)	phensuximide (Milontin)
phenytoin (Dilantin)	**Other Drugs**
Oxazolidinediones	acetazolamide (Diamox)
paramethadione (Paradione)	bromides
carbamazepine (Tegretol)	carbamazepine (Tegretol)
trimethadione (Tridione)	corticotropin (ACTH) and corticosteroids
	dextroamphetamine (Dexedrine)
	phenacemide (Phenurone)
	quinacrine (Atabrine)
	valproic acid (Depakene)

[a] Primidone is a deoxybarbiturate.

ested in rarely prescribed agents or in detailed coverage of the medical management of epilepsy are referred to the sources listed as selected readings for this chapter.

Tonic-Clonic Seizures

At one time, phenytoin, phenobarbital, and primidone were the agents most often used to treat generalized tonic-clonic (grand mal) seizures. Phenytoin was generally favored with adults, phenobarbital with children. In recent years, however, carbamazepine and even valproic acid have come to be seen as drugs of first choice by many physicians who specialize in the treatment of epilepsy.

Absence Seizures

Ethosuximide, valproic acid, and clonazepam are the agents most often used to treat absence (petit mal) seizures.

Partial Seizures

Drugs used to treat tonic-clonic seizures also are used to control simple partial seizures and complex partial seizures. Of them, carbamazepine is generally preferred. Phenytoin, phenobarbital, and primidone are also used but are less popular than in previous decades. Valproic acid may be of value in controlling complex partial seizures, especially when combined with other agents.

Seizures in Infants and Young Children

Usual antiepileptic medications are typically ineffective in treating infantile spasms with hypsarrhythmia. Corticotropins and adrenocorticotropins are the drugs of choice for this difficult-to-manage condition. Valproic acid appears to be the drug of choice in managing myoclonic epilepsy (DeVito, 1983) in very young people. Clonazepam is also sometimes useful.

BEHAVIORAL AND PHYSIOLOGICAL ACTIONS OF ANTIEPILEPTIC DRUGS

The precise biochemical mechanisms through which specific antiepileptic drugs produce their effects are poorly understood and are not addressed here. In general, these drugs can reduce seizures in two ways (Rall & Schleifer, 1985). One is by preventing or attenuating the excessive electrical activity of neurons at focal sites where seizures are initiated. The other is by preventing the spread of electrical activity from focal sites to surrounding neurons. Because all antiepileptic medications currently used reduce the ability of the brain to respond to seizure-provoking stimuli, they appear to act at least in part through this second mechanism.

Antiepileptic medications have a wide range of actions in addition to the ability to control seizures and for this reason induce a variety of side effects, some of which are troublesome—so troublesome, in fact, that a major goal in the pharmacological management of epilepsy is choosing a drug and dosage regimen that adequately controls seizures without causing intolerable side effects.

The kind and severity of side effects depend upon the agent in question and the dose at which it is administered. Drugs with similar chemical structures may differ significantly with respect to side effects, and the agent that produces fewer or milder side effects is generally preferred. For example, both phenytoin and mephenytoin reduce tonic-clonic and psychomotor seizures, but the serious and potentially life-threatening side effects of mephenytoin, including aplastic anemia (reduced red blood cells) and pancytopenia (reduction in all cellular elements of the blood), render phenytoin preferable. Unfortunately, phenytoin also produces a range of undesirable side effects, including nausea, vomiting, skin rashes, excessive growth of the gums (gingival hyperplasia), headache, excessive hair growth (hirsutism), confusion, and learning impairment.

Side effects of antiepileptic drugs can in general be classified as (a) toxic effects due to inappropriately high drug blood levels, (b) common side effects that appear at therapeutic blood levels, and (c) so-called idiosyncratic effects that are not closely related to blood levels. These latter effects are not truly idiosyncratic, but rather uncommon side effects that appear in a small proportion of treated individuals. In general, with all antiepileptics the risk and severity of side effects increases with dosage.

At very low doses, an antiepileptic drug typically produces few undesirable side effects, but therapeutic effects are also absent. As the dose increases, the proportion of patients demonstrating a therapeutic response grows, but the proportion experiencing troublesome side effects does the same until, when toxic levels are reached, adverse reactions are observed in all treated individuals. Antiepileptic drugs are of therapeutic value only at doses that control seizures without inducing intolerable side effects. The range of doses likely to do so is established through the study of many individuals with epilepsy and is called the suggested optimal therapeutic level (SOTL) (Gibbs et al., 1982). SOTLs have been established for all of the commonly used antiepileptics. These levels are not expressed in terms of amount of drug taken but in terms of the amount of medication in the blood. Drug blood level is a better measure than absolute dosage because people differ widely with respect to rates of absorption, biotransformation, and excretion of anticonvulsant drugs. In addition, the rate of metabolism of many antiepileptics varies with dosage, and several anticonvulsants are biotransformed to active metabolites that have seizure-reducing properties. For these reasons, the oral doses required to reach SOTLs vary widely across individuals, are not a very good predictor of therapeutic response, and can only be specified within a broad range. Table 8.3 lists, for several antiepileptic drugs, characteristic oral dose ranges and therapeutic blood levels in children. Doses and therapeutic blood levels characteristically are similar or higher in adults.

Because a few individuals experience adequate seizure control at drug blood levels below the SOTL and some experience significant side effects within this range, SOTLs are not intended to be rigid limits within which all patients must be maintained. Rather, early in treatment, the physician uses the SOTL as a target to be reached through rapid titration of dosage. Once drug blood levels are within the SOTL, they can be adjusted upward or downward, always with the goal of providing adequate seizure control and minimal side effects.

In the everyday management of epilepsy, medication is administered orally, and an attempt is made to space dosings so that stable drug blood levels are obtained across time. Ensuring constant drug blood levels is necessary both to control seizures and to avert toxic drug effects. There is controversy as to the appropriate schedule of administration for various antiepileptic drugs. For example, some clinicians argue that convenience dictates that phenytoin and phenobarbital should

Table 8.3. Pharmacological Properties of Selected Antiepileptic Drugs in Children

Drug	Usual Dose (mg/kg/day)	Therapeutic Blood Levels (μg/ml)	Time to Stable Blood Level
carbamazepine	10–15	6–12	2–4 days
clonazepam	0.05–0.2	20–80 (ng/ml)	4–12 days
ethosuximide	15–35	40–100	6–12 days
phenobarbital	4–6	15–40	8–15 days
phenytoin	5–10	10–20	2–5 days
primidone	12–25	5–10	20–30 hours
valproic acid	15–60	50–100	30–75 hours

Note: All values are as reported by Gadow (1986b)

be administered only once per day. Others (e.g., Livingston, 1978), however, suggest that these drugs typically should be administered in two or three divided dosings each day so as to produce stable blood levels, with once-a-day schedules of administration used only when blood level studies and clinical observations support their utility. Many patients for whom phenytoin or phenobarbital are prescribed take these agents in two or three divided doses per day, but others do well with a single daily administration. With the exception of valproic acid, which has a short half-life, antiepileptic medications typically need to be taken no more often than twice a day; and once-a-day administration will suffice for many patients (Gibbs et al., 1982).

Regardless of whether an antiepileptic drug is to be taken once a day or more often, patients must receive the drug at the scheduled time and dose. Patient noncompliance is a major cause of unstable drug blood levels, and it has been reported that approximately 50% of outpatients with poorly controlled seizures failed to take their medications as intended by their physicians (Gibbs et al., 1982). Ensuring that drugs are taken at the intended time and dosage is an important goal for the nursing staff and others who deal with this population.

It must be recognized that a considerable period of time is required for drug blood levels to stabilize when an antiepileptic drug is first administered or when dosage is altered. In general, the time required for blood levels to stabilize varies directly with the half-life of the drug. For example, stable drug blood levels of phenytoin (which has a half-life of 18 to 30 hours) are reached within 1 to 2 weeks, whereas 3 to 4 weeks may be necessary for blood levels of phenobarbital (which has a half-life of 50 to 120 hours) to stabilize.

ASSESSING THERAPEUTIC AND SIDE EFFECTS OF ANTIEPILEPTIC MEDICATIONS

Information concerning the frequency of seizures and the severity of side effects is necessary to evaluate an antiepileptic medication regimen. When mentally deficient or nonverbal people receive such drugs, caregivers should work closely with physicians to make certain that such information is collected accurately. With patients who are able to describe their own physical and behavioral status, self-reports play an important role in detecting adverse reactions to medication. For example, a patient who begins receiving phenobarbital to control tonic-clonic seizures may report that, in the third week of treatment, no seizures occurred, but the drug produced pronounced and vexing drowsiness. This is a relatively common side effect of phenobarbital, one to which tolerance frequently develops. Thus, the physician might ask the patient to continue taking the same dose for a few more weeks in the hope that drowsiness would abate while seizure control continued. Self-report data would determine whether this occurred. If drowsiness continued to be a problem, alteration of treatment, perhaps in the form of a reduction in dosage, would be in order.

When patients are not able to report on side effects, as frequently occurs with severely and profoundly mentally retarded patients, care must be taken to ensure that they are not overmedicated. Drug-induced physiological changes usually can be detected by conventional medical examinations, but behavioral toxicity, such as disruption of learning, can be detected only by direct observation. Although there are no standardized procedures for measuring behavioral and cognitive side effects of antiepileptic medications, a growing body of literature suggests that most if not all antiepileptic medications can in some situations deleteriously affect learning and performance of desired behaviors (e.g., Gadow, 1986). In view of this, measures that reflect these dimensions should be closely monitored.

Caregivers should also be alert to the wide range of deleterious physiological side effects of antiepileptic drugs and ask physicians what reactions might occur and how to detect them. For example, blood disorders may be associated with sore throat, fever, easy bruising, nosebleed, weakness, and hemorrhage made apparent by red or purple spots on the skin. Because some side effects are not easily detected by observation alone, regular physical and laboratory tests (which will vary in nature and frequency depending upon the specific medication involved) must be arranged.

The following is a listing of some of the side effects associated with various antiepileptic drugs and a summary of their clinical applications. It must be recognized that this list is not exhaustive and that unduly high blood levels of all antiepileptic drugs produce toxic effects that may differ in kind and intensity from side effects observed at therapeutic levels.

Barbiturates

The barbiturates are commonly used antiepileptic medications generally effective in treating tonic-clonic and complex partial seizures. Drowsiness is a common side effect of phenobarbital (and other barbiturates). In children, drug-induced behavior problems (hyperactivity, irritability, aggression, and excitability) also occur frequently. These behavior problems, which are not dose-related, may in some cases be more troublesome than an occasional seizure. In some cases, concurrent treatment with methylphenidate or dextroamphetamine reduces phenobarbital-induced behavioral disturbances (Livingston, 1978). Phenobarbital sometimes produces confusion in elderly patients.

Phenobarbital has been associated with several other side effects, most of low prevalence. Among them are nausea and vomiting, dizziness, blood disorders, and headache.

Metharbital (Gemonil) appears to have greater sedative and weaker antiepileptic action than phenobarbital. Its use is largely restricted to the treatment of infantile spasms and to children who become hyperactive on phenobarbital. Side effects are similar to those of phenobarbital.

Primidone appears to produce its actions through two active metabolities, phenobarbital and phenylethylmalonamide. Side effects associated with primidone are sedation, headaches, dizziness, vertigo, nausea, double vision, and rapid involuntary eye movements (nystagmus). Rashes, blood disorders, inflammatory disturbances (systemic lupus erythematosus), and disturbances of lymphatic function have been reported but are rare. Hyperactivity is not a major problem with primidone, but acute psychotic reactions do occasionally occur, usually in patients with complex partial epilepsy. Like many other antiepileptic drugs, primidone occasionally interferes with folate and vitamin D utilization.

Benzodiazepines

Clonazepam is the benzodiazepine most often used to manage seizures. It is valuable in treating absence (petit mal) seizures and myoclonic seizures in children. The primary side effects of the drug are drowsiness, fatigue, and lethargy. Muscle incoordination and ataxia (failure of muscular coordination) appear less often, as do dizziness, speech impairment, and increased salivary and bronchial secretions. Behavioral disturbances (e.g., aggression, irritability, hyperactivity, and reduced attention span) have also been reported. Severe drowsiness occurs in nearly half of the individuals treated with clonazepam, ataxia in about a third, and a quarter exhibit behavioral disturbance (aggressivity, irritability, hyperactivity, and agitation) (Gadow, 1986). Because some patients with the types of seizures (myoclonic and akinetic) for which clonazepam is recommended are severely mentally retarded, the adverse effects of the drug on the patient's ability to perform personal tasks, walk, or communicate may outweigh the benefit of controlling seizures.

Diazepam is prescribed primarily for the treatment of status epilepticus (where the drug is given by slow intravenous injection) and myoclonic seizures. Its side effects are similar to those of clonazepam.

Hydantoins

Phenytoin is the most commonly prescribed hydantoin. Like the other hydantoins (ethotoin and mephenytoin), it is useful in treating all types of epilepsy except absence seizures. Phenytoin often does not produce drowsiness at therapeutic levels, but the drug can in some cases deleteriously affect learning and adaptive behavior. Ataxia, double vision, hallucinations, dizziness, and changes in behavior (e.g., hyperactivity, confusion) occur at toxic doses, but these untoward effects are generally alleviated by dosage reduction. Excessive growth of the gum tissue (gingival hyperplasia) occurs in a sizeable minority (c. 30%) of patients treated with phenytoin. Good oral hygiene can prevent problems associated with food trapped in the enlarged gums, but it cannot slow or prevent growth of gum tissue, which slowly returns to normal size following drug discontinuation. Hirsutism (excessive hair growth), occurs in some individuals treated with phenytoin and may pose a real problem for certain women. Phenytoin sometimes produces stomach pain, nausea, and anorexia (loss of appetite); these effects usually can be lessened by taking the drug with meals or in several small divided doses. Constipation is occasionally a problem with chronic phenytoin use, as is peripheral neuropathy, which can interfere with tendon reflexes and is most common in elderly patients. Other side effects of phenytoin, all of which are rare, include hyperglycemia, blood disorders, rashes, and coarse facies, a thickening of the skin of the nose, mouth, and forehead.

Mephenytoin (Mesantoin) has the same clinical applications as phenytoin and is less likely to produce ataxia, gingival hyperplasia, gastric distress, hirsutism, or sedation. Mephenytoin is, however, associated with a range of serious side effects, including fever, morbid changes in the lymph nodes, measles-like rashes, and a variety of blood disorders. These actions limit its usefulness.

Though its side effects are minimal, ethotoin (Peganone) is only mildly effective in controlling seizures and therefore is typically used in combination with other antiepileptic drugs. Adverse effects include rashes, drowsiness, double vision, nausea, headache, and ataxia.

Succinimides

The succinimides (ethosuximide, methsuximide, and phensuximide) are used primarily to manage absence seizures. Ethosuximide is the best-studied of these agents. Its reported side effects include gastrointestinal complaints (nausea, vomiting, anorexia), drowsiness, lethargy, dizziness, lupus-like disorders, headache, skin rashes, hiccups, and behavioral disturbances involving restlessness, agitation, anxiety, and aggression. Behavioral disturbances are most common in patients with a history of psychiatric disorder (Rall & Schleifer, 1985). Blood dyscrasias are a significant side effect of succinimides, and in a small number of patients they have proven fatal. Hence, when patients receive ethosuximide, "it is generally recommended that periodic blood counts be performed at no greater than monthly intervals for the duration of treatment and that the dosage be reduced or the drug discontinued should the total white blood count fall below 3,500 or the proportion of granulocytes below 25% of the total white blood count" (Dreifuss, 1982, p. 650).

Side effects of methsuximide (Celontin) and phensuximide (Milontin) have not been studied carefully. These drugs are reported to produce, in some individuals, central nervous system and gastrointestinal effects similar to those associated with ethosuximide (i.e., nausea, anorexia, headaches, hiccups, drowsiness, and dizziness).

Oxazolidinediones

Paramethadione (Paradione) and trimethadione (Tridione) were once commonly used for treating absence seizures but are rarely prescribed today. The actions of the two agents are very similar, but the latter is more often used and has been more carefully studied. Day blindness and photophobia are the most prevalent side effects of these drugs, and are observed in a significant minority of patients. When photophobia is present, visual acuity decreases as illumination increases and bright lights are perceived as irritating. Tolerance often develops to photophobia, and dark glasses can be worn to minimize its impact. Other adverse effects include headache, drowsiness, skin rashes, nausea, hiccups, abdominal pain, double vision, ataxia, restlessness, weight loss, decreased concentration, dizziness, and fatigue. Insomnia, restlessness, confusion, and hallucinations are observed in some patients. Depressed function of kidneys and bone marrow are serious but rare side effects of trimethadione and paramethadione.

Other Drugs

Carbamazepine, used alone and in combination with other drugs, is of value in managing complex partial and tonic-clonic seizures. Relatively common side effects of carbamazepine are neurotoxic reactions involving double or blurred vision, drowsiness, dizziness, nausea and vomiting, slurred speech, and ataxia. Treatment with carbamazepine has been associated with psychotic behavior, hyperactivity, water retention, and various forms of involuntary movement disorders. By depressing bone marrow function, carbamazepine can produce a variety of serious hematological (blood) disorders. Although rare, these disorders are serious to the point of being life-threatening. Because of this, laboratory analyses of hematological function are necessary for patients receiving carbamazepine.

Valproic acid is most often prescribed for the control of absence seizures; it is also of some value in treating tonic-clonic and myoclonic seizures. Gastrointestinal symptoms such as anorexia, nausea, and vomiting are the most common adverse side effects of valproic acid. They can often be reduced by administering the enteric-coated form of the drug. Other reported side effects are tremor, irritability, aggressiveness, sleep disturbances, hair thinning, liver disorders (including toxic hepatitis), and pancreatitis. Liver disorders associated with valproic acid have been fatal in several cases, most involving children and patients with intractable epilepsy, often accompanied by mental retardation. These disorders usually occur within 6 months of treatment, and it is crucial to carefully monitor hepatic function during this period. Moreover, the drug should be withdrawn immediately whenever clinical symptoms of drowsiness, lethargy, loss of seizure control, or gastrointestinal upset is observed, for these symptoms have preceded fatal responses to the drug (Jeavons, 1982).

Teratogenesis and Antiepileptic Drugs

Prescription of antiepileptic medications to pregnant women raises the issue of possible harm to the developing fetus. Although most (>90% of) epileptic women treated with antiepileptic drugs who become pregnant bear normal children (Rall & Schleifer, 1985), their risk of bearing children with birth defects is 1.25 to 2 times as great as for nonepileptic women (Bossi, 1983). It is not clear whether the antiepileptic drugs cause major or minor birth defects, because the incidence of defects is also elevated in epileptic women who do not take medication during pregnancy (Bossi, 1983). Phenytoin was once thought to produce a characteristic pattern of congenital malformations (termed the fetal hydantoin syndrome), but this does not appear to be the case (Shapiro et al., 1976). Information concerning possible teratogenic effects of specific antiepileptic medications is provided by Woodbury et al. (1982).

ADVERSE EFFECTS OF WITHDRAWING ANTIEPILEPTIC MEDICATIONS

Some individuals who receive antiepileptic drugs and have been seizure-free for a period of time can be withdrawn from medication. The likelihood of this occurring is greatest in children whose seizures began early in life and were rapidly and easily controlled. A general rule for the discontinuation of medication for seizure disorders is to wait at least 4 years after the last seizure before considering the termination of medication (Livingston, 1972, 1978). Withdrawal of medication should involve a very gradual reduction of dosage, for sudden termination of treatment is likely to precipitate seizure activity.

DRUG INTERACTIONS

As noted previously, the concurrent prescription of two or more antiepileptic drugs is commonplace. Moreover, individuals receiving antiepileptic medication frequently take other kinds of drugs. In general, interactions between antiepileptic drugs involve changes in the rate of drug biotransformation, frequently through enzyme induction or inhibition (see chapter 2). For example, when phenytoin is given to a person receiving carbamazepine, inactivation of carbamazepine is enhanced through phenytoin-induced increases in the enzymes that break down carbamazepines. And, unless dosages are raised, carbamazepine blood levels fall.

Detailed coverage of how specific antiepileptic drugs interact with one another and with other drugs is provided by Woodbury et al. (1982), whose text is an excellent reference. Nonmedical personnel who care for epileptic individuals need only to be aware that drug interactions can and do occur. Therefore, whenever there is a change in the kind or amount of medication that an epileptic person is receiving, any change in seizure frequency or adverse side effect should be promptly reported to the appropriate health care provider.

TREATMENT DURING SEIZURES

Even when medication is used appropriately, some epileptic patients have seizures at least occasionally. Once a seizure has started, there is nothing that can be done to stop it. Unless momentary loss of consciousness creates a dangerous situation, absence and psychomotor seizures dictate no intervention by care providers. In the case of tonic-clonic seizures, the following guidelines may prove useful.

1. Remain calm. Seizures characteristically are not dangerous in and of themselves.

2. Clear the area around the individual to prevent self-injury. When potentially harmful objects cannot be moved, use your body to shield the person from them. If in a wheelchair, the person should be eased to the floor. Place him or her prone or lying on one side, and turn the head to one side to allow saliva to drain easily. A soft object can be placed under the head as a pillow, but this is not necessary. If a pillow is used, it should not force the head forward.

3. Do not try to restrain the individual, to restrict motions in any way, or to place anything between the teeth.

4. Remove food, gum, and vomitus from the mouth, and make sure that the mouth and nose are uncovered so that breathing is unobstructed. *A primary goal in dealing with seizures is to allow free breathing.*

5. Remove or loosen tight clothing.

6. Remain with the individual until the seizure ceases. Do not try to revive the person with water, by shaking, or in any other way.

7. Once consciousness returns, a small child (if it seems advisable) can be carried to a private area. Larger individuals should be allowed to retire to a private area to sleep and rest for a time if they so desire.

8. Recognize that the individual is not responsible for his or her actions during the course of a seizure and deal with the incident in a matter-of-fact way.

9. Caregivers should record each incident of seizure activity in their charges.

10. Prolonged seizures or seizures that repeat serially require prompt medical attention (usually involving the intravenous administration of diazepam or a barbiturate).

If one or more incidents of apparent seizure activity are observed in an individual not known to be an epileptic, caregivers should accurately record relevant information about the incident. To aid medical personnel in determining whether an individual is actually having seizures, the following information should be recorded:

1. When and where did the seizure occur? What was happening prior to the seizure?

2. Did the individual engage in any unusual behavior (e.g., cry out) before the seizure?

3. What kinds of movements occurred during the seizure? Were movements generalized or confined to one side of the body? If a number of movements were observed, in what sequence did they occur? Accurate reporting may be facilitated by providing specific descriptions of movements (if any) of the eyes, head, arms and hands, facial muscles, legs, and trunk.

4. Did the individual urinate or defecate during the seizure?

5. What was the duration of the seizure?

6. How did the individual behave after the seizure?

7. Was the seizure preceded by an aura? If so, what was its nature? Did the individual verbally report the aura prior to the seizure or recall its presence after the incident?

8. Was the person obviously ill, stressed, or fatigued prior to the seizure? It is especially important to note whether the individual had a fever at or before the incident.

In educational, treatment, and residential settings where seizures are likely to occur, specific procedures for dealing with seizures and recording their occurrences should be developed and all staff members familiarized with them. Attending physicians and the epileptic patients themselves, when appropriate, should play major roles in developing these procedures.

CONCLUDING COMMENT

Millions of people with epilepsy have had their seizures controlled with medication, allowing them to lead essentially normal lives. An important concern in the pharmacological management of epilepsy is arranging a drug regimen that minimizes adverse reactions, including disruption of learning, memory, and performance, while providing adequate seizure control. This issue is especially important with respect to patients who are not able to report side effects.

Appendix A
List of Selected Drugs by Generic (Nonproprietary) Name

Generic Name	Trade Name[a]	Classification
acetazolamide	Diamox	antiepileptic, diuretic
acetophenazine	Tindal	antipsychotic
alprozolam	Xanax	antianxiety
amatadine	Symmetrel	antiparkinsonian
amitryptyline	Elavil, Endep	antidepressant
amobarbital	Amytal	sedative, hypnotic
amoxapine	Asendin	antidepressant
amphetamine	Benzedrine	stimulant
aprobarbital	Alurate	sedative, hypnotic
benztropine	Cogentin	anticholinergic, antiparkinsonian
biperiden	Akineton	anticholinergic, antiparkinsonian
buspirone	BuSpar	antianxiety
butabarbital	Butisol	sedative, hypnotic
carbamazepine	Tegretol	antiepileptic
chloral hydrate	Noctec	sedative, hypnotic
chloridazepoxide	Librium	antianxiety
chlormezanone	Trancopal	antianxiety
chlorpromazine	Thorazine	antipsychotic
chlorprothixene	Taractan	antipsychotic
clomipramine	Not approved[b]	antidepressant
clonazepam	Klonopin	antiepileptic
clonidine	Catapres	antihypertensive
clorazepate	Tranxene	antianxiety

149

Generic Name	Trade Name[a]	Classification
cyproheptadine	Periactin	antiasthmatic
dantrolene sodium	Dantrium	skeletal muscle relaxant
deanol	Deaner	stimulant
desipramine	Norpramin, Pertofrane	antidepressant
desmethylimipramine	Not approved	antidepressant
dextroamphetamine	Dexedrine	stimulant
diazepam	Valium	antiepileptic, skeletal muscle relaxant, antianxiety
diphenhydramine	Benadryl	sedative, hypnotic, antihistamine
diphenylhydantoin	Dilantin	antiepileptic
doxepin	Adapin, Sinequan	antidepressant
ethchlorvynol	Placidyl	sedative, hypnotic
ethimate	Valmid	sedative, hypnotic
ethopropazine	Parsidol	anticholinergic, antiparkinsonian
ethosuximide	Zarontin	antiepileptic
ethotoin	Peganone	antiepileptic
fenfluramine	Pondimin	anorectic
fluoxetine	Prozac	antidepressant
fluphenazine	Prolixin, Permitil	antipsychotic
flurazepam	Dalmane	sedative, hypnotic
glutethimide	Doriden	sedative, hypnotic
halazepam	Paxipam	antianxiety
haloperidol	Haldol	antipsychotic
hydroxyzine	Atarax, Vistaril, Durrax	sedative, hypnotic, antianxiety
imipramine	Janimine, SK-Pramine, Tofranil	antidepressant
isocarboxazid	Marplan	antidepressant
levoamphetamine	Not approved	stimulant
lithium carbonate	Eskalith, Lithane, Lithonate	antipsychotic
lorazepam	Ativan	antianxiety
loxapine	Loxitane	antipsychotic
maprotiline	Ludiomil	antidepressant
mephenytoin	Mesantoin	antiepileptic
mephobarbital	Mebaral	antiepileptic
meprobamate	Miltown, Equanil	antianxiety
mesoridazine	Serentil	antipsychotic

Generic Name	Trade Name[a]	Classification
methamphetamine	Desoxyn	stimulant
methaqualone	Quaalude, Sopor	sedative, hypnotic
metharbital	Gemontil	antiepileptic
methsuximide	Celontin	antiepileptic
methylphenidate	Ritalin	stimulant
methyprylon	Noludar	sedative, hypnotic
molindone	Moban	antipsychotic
nomifensine	Merital	antidepressant
nortriptyline	Aventyl, Pamelor	antidepressant
oxazepan	Serax	antianxiety
paramethadione	Paradione	antiepileptic
pemoline	Cylert	stimulant
penfluridol	Not approved	antipsychotic
pentobarbital	Nembutal	sedative, hypnotic
perphenazine	Trilafon	antipsychotic
phenacemide	Phenurone	antiepileptic
phenelzine	Nardil	antidepressant
phenobarbital	Luminal	antiepileptic, sedative, hypnotic
phensuximide	Milontin	antiepileptic
phenytoin	Dilantin	antiepileptic
pimozide	Orap	antipsychotic
piperacetazine	Quide	antipsychotic
prazepam	Centrax	antianxiety
primidone	Mysoline	antiepileptic
prochlorperazine	Compazine	antipsychotic
procyclidine	Kemadrin	anticholinergic, antiparkinsonian
promazine	Sparine	antipsychotic
promethazine	Phenergan	sedative, hypnotic
propranolol	Inderal	beta-adrenergic blocker
protriptyline	Vivactil	antidepressant
quinacrine	Atabrine	antiparkinsonian
reserpine	Serapsil	antipsychotic
secobarbital	Seconal	sedative, hypnotic
temazepam	Restoril	sedative, hypnotic
thioridazine	Mellaril	antipsychotic
thiothixene	Navane	antipsychotic
tranylcypromine	Parnate	antidepressant
trazodone	Desyrel	antidepressant
triazolam	Halcion	sedative, hypnotic

Generic Name	Trade Name[a]	Classification
trifluoperazine	Stelazine	antipsychotic
triflupromazine	Vesprin	antipsychotic
trihexyphenidyl	Artane	anticholinergic, antiparkin-soniam
trimethadione	Trione	antiepileptic
trimipramine	Surmontil	antidepressant
valproic acid	Depakene	antiepileptic

[a] For drugs no longer protected by patent laws, the inclusion of trade names other than the original was arbitrary.
[b] Drugs listed as "Not Approved" were not approved for general use by the Food and Drug Administration as of 1988.

Appendix B

Monitoring of Side-Effects System (Moses)

Client: _____	SCALE		
ID #: _____	0 = Not present	3 = Moderate	
Date: _____	1 = Minimal	4 = Severe	
Rater: _____	2 = Mild	NA = Not Assessed	

EYES/EARS

1. Blurred vision	0	1	2	3	4	5	NA
2. Double vision	0	1	2	3	4	5	NA
3. Eyes rolled up	0	1	2	3	4	5	NA
4. Movement: rapid vertical/horizontal	0	1	2	3	4	5	NA
5. Ringing in ears	0	1	2	3	4	5	NA

GASTROINTESTINAL, INCLUDING MOUTH

6. Abdominal pain/cramps	0	1	2	3	4	5	NA
7. Appetite: decreased/anorexia	0	1	2	3	4	5	NA
8. Appetite: increased	0	1	2	3	4	5	NA
9. Constipation	0	1	2	3	4	5	NA
10. Diarrhea	0	1	2	3	4	5	NA
11. Drooling/salivation	0	1	2	3	4	5	NA
12. Dry mouth	0	1	2	3	4	5	NA
13. Gas/indigestion	0	1	2	3	4	5	NA
14. Gum growth	0	1	2	3	4	5	NA
15. Nausea	0	1	2	3	4	5	NA
16. Taste: abnormal/metallic	0	1	2	3	4	5	NA
17. Thirst: increased	0	1	2	3	4	5	NA
18. Vomiting	0	1	2	3	4	5	NA

NEUROLOGICAL/MUSCLE

19. Contortions/spasticity	0	1	2	3	4	5	NA
20. Gait: imbalance/unsteady	0	1	2	3	4	5	NA
21. Gait: shuffling	0	1	2	3	4	5	NA
22. Headache	0	1	2	3	4	5	NA
23. Inability to sit still/pacing/ restlessness	0	1	2	3	4	5	NA
24. Limb jerking/writhing	0	1	2	3	4	5	NA
25. Lip smacking/chewing/tongue movements/grimacing	0	1	2	3	4	5	NA
26. Mask-like, expressionless face	0	1	2	3	4	5	NA
27. Neck/back arching	0	1	2	3	4	5	NA
28. Pill rolling	0	1	2	3	4	5	NA
29. Rigidity	0	1	2	3	4	5	NA
30. Slurred speech	0	1	2	3	4	5	NA
31. Tremor	0	1	2	3	4	5	NA

PSYCHOLOGICAL/GENERAL

32. Agitation/jitters	0	1	2	3	4	5	NA
33. Anxiety	0	1	2	3	4	5	NA
34. Attention/concentration: decrease	0	1	2	3	4	5	NA
35. Confusion	0	1	2	3	4	5	NA
36. Depression	0	1	2	3	4	5	NA
37. Drowsiness/sedation	0	1	2	3	4	5	NA
38. Irritability	0	1	2	3	4	5	NA
39. Lethargy/no movement	0	1	2	3	4	5	NA
40. Psychosis: hallucinations/etc.	0	1	2	3	4	5	NA
41. Sleep: excessive	0	1	2	3	4	5	NA
42. Sleep: insomnia/less	0	1	2	3	4	5	NA
43. Weakness/fatigue	0	1	2	3	4	5	NA

RESPIRATORY

44. Difficult/labored breathing	0	1	2	3	4	5	NA
45. Nasal congestion	0	1	2	3	4	5	NA

SKIN

46. Acne	0	1	2	3	4	5	NA
47. Abnormal hair growth	0	1	2	3	4	5	NA
48. Color: pale/pallor	0	1	2	3	4	5	NA
49. Color: yellow	0	1	2	3	4	5	NA
50. Itching/dry	0	1	2	3	4	5	NA
51. Puffy/tissue fluid	0	1	2	3	4	5	NA
52. Rash/hives	0	1	2	3	4	5	NA

| 53. Sunburn/photosensitivity | 0 | 1 | 2 | 3 | 4 | 5 | NA |
| 54. Sweating: increased | 0 | 1 | 2 | 3 | 4 | 5 | NA |

URINARY

55. Breast: swelling/growth	0	1	2	3	4	5	NA
56. Breast: discharge	0	1	2	3	4	5	NA
57. Menstrual: absence	0	1	2	3	4	5	NA
58. Menstrual: irregularities	0	1	2	3	4	5	NA
59. Sexual: decreased/impotence	0	1	2	3	4	5	NA
60. Sexual: increased	0	1	2	3	4	5	NA
61. Urinary: decreased/retention	0	1	2	3	4	5	NA
62. Urinary: difficult/painful	0	1	2	3	4	5	NA
63. Urinary: enuresis/nocturesis	0	1	2	3	4	5	NA
64. Urinary: increased	0	1	2	3	4	5	NA

WHOLE BODY

65. Convulsions/seizures	0	1	2	3	4	5	NA
66. Fainting/dizziness	0	1	2	3	4	5	NA
67. Fever	0	1	2	3	4	5	NA
68. Sore throat	0	1	2	3	4	5	NA
69. Weight: gain	0	1	2	3	4	5	NA
70. Weight: loss	0	1	2	3	4	5	NA

MEASURES
71. Blood Pressure: —— / ——
72. Pulse: ——
73. Weight: —— lbs

OTHER

74. ———————————————	0	1	2	3	4	5	NA
75. ———————————————	0	1	2	3	4	5	NA
76. ———————————————	0	1	2	3	4	5	NA
77. ———————————————	0	1	2	3	4	5	NA

Note: Assessment sheet for Monitoring of Side-Effects System (MOSES). Copyright 1986 by J. E. Kalachnik. Reprinted with permission.

References

Abikoff, H., Gittelman-Klein, R. & Klein, D. F. (1977). Validation of a classroom observation code for hyperactive children. *Journal of Consulting and Clinical Psychology, 45,*
772–783.

Addonizio, G. (1985). Rapid induction of extrapyramidal side effects with combined use
of lithium and neuroleptics. *Journal of Clinical Psychopharmacology, 5,* 296–298.

Aman, M. G. (1978). Drugs, learning and the psychotherapies. In J. S. Werry (ed.),
Pediatric psychopharmacology: The use of behavior modifying drugs in children (pp. 79–108).
New York: Brunner/Mazel.

Aman, M. G. & Singh, N. N. (1983). Pharmacological interventions. In J. A. Matson &
J. A. Mulick (Eds.), *Handbook of mental retardation* (pp. 317–338). Elmsford, NY: Pergamon Press.

Aman, M. G., Field, C. J. & Bridgman, G. D. (1985). City-wide survey of drug patterns
among non-institutionalized mentally retarded persons. *Applied Research in Mental Retardation, 6,* 159–171.

Aman, M. G., Singh, N. N., Steward, A. W. & Field, C. J. (1985). The Aberrant Behavior
Checklist: A behavior rating scale for the assessment of treatment effects. *American
Journal of Mental Deficiency, 89,* 485–491.

Ambrosini, P. J. (1987). Pharmacotherapy in child and adolescent major depressive disorder. In H. Y. Meltzer (Ed.), *Psychopharmacology: The third generation of progress* (pp.
1247–1254). New York: Raven Press.

Amdisen, A. (1969). Variation of serum lithium concentration during the day in relation
to treatment control, absorptive side-effects, and the use of slow-release tablets. *Acta
Psychiatrica Scandinavica, 207,* 55–58.

American Psychiatric Association. (1987). *Diagnostic and statistical manual of mental disorders (3rd ed. rev.).* Washington, DC: Author.

Anderson, L. T., Campbell, M., Grega, D. M., Perry, R., Small, A. M. & Green, W. H.
(1984). Haloperidol in the treatment of infantile autism: Effects on learning and behavioral symptoms. *American Journal of Psychiatry, 141,* 1195–1202.

Arana, G. W., Goff, D. C., Baldessarini, R. J. & Keepers, G. A. (1988). Efficacy of anticholinergic prophylaxis for neuroleptic-induced acute dystonia. *American Journal of Psychiatry, 145,* 993–996.

Association of Professional Sleep Societies. (1987). *Diagnostic classification of sleep and arousal
disorders.* Rochester, MN: Author.

Atre-Vaidya, N. & Taylor, M. A. (1989). Effectiveness of lithium in schizophrenia: Do we
really have an answer? *Journal of Clinical Psychiatry, 50,* 170–173.

Avorn, J., Dreyer, P., Connelly, K. & Soumerai, S. B. (1989). Use of psychoactive medication and the quality of care in rest homes. *New England Journal of Medicine, 320,* 227–232.

Ayd, F. J. (1961). A survey of drug-induced extrapyramidal reactions. *Journal of the American Medical Association, 175,* 1054–1060.

Baldessarini, R. J. (1985a). *Chemotherapy in psychiatry.* Cambridge, MA: Harvard University Press.

Baldessarini, R. J. (1985b). Drugs and the treatment of psychiatric disorders. In A. G. Gilman, L. S. Goodman, T. W. Rall & F. Murad (Eds.). *The pharmacological basis of therapeutics* (pp. 387–446). New York: Macmillan.

Baldessarini, R. J. (1989). Current status of antidepressants: Clinical pharmacology and therapy. *Journal of Clinical Psychiatry, 50,* 117–126.

Baldessarini, R. J., Cohen, B. M. & Teicher, M. H. (1988). Significance of neuroleptic dose and plasma level in the pharmacological treatment of psychoses. *Archives of General Psychiatry, 45,* 79–91.

Baldessarini, R. J., Katz, B. & Cotton, P. (1984). Dissimilar dosing with high-potency and low-potency neuroleptics. *American Journal of Psychiatry, 141,* 748–752.

Barkley, R. A. (1977). A review of stimulant drug research with hyperactive children. *Journal of Child Psychology and Psychiatry, 18,* 137–165.

Barkley, R. A. (1981). *Hyperactive children: A handbook for diagnosis and treatment.* New York: Guilford Press.

Barkley, R. A. & Cunningham, C. E. (1978). Do stimulant drugs improve the academic performance of hyperactive children? *Clinical Pediatrics, 17,* 85–92.

Barkley, R. A., Karlsson, J., Strzelecki, E. & Murphy, J. V. (1984). Effects of age and Ritalin dosage on the mother–child interactions of hyperactive children. *Journal of Consulting and Clinical Psychology, 52,* 750–758.

Barnes, T. R. E. & Braude, W. M. (1985). Akathisia variants and tardive dyskinesia. *Archives of General Psychiatry, 42,* 874–878.

Bauer, A. M. & Shea, T. M. (1984). Tourette syndrome: A review and educational implications. *Journal of Autism and Developmental Disorders, 14,* 69–80.

Beresford, R. & Ward, A. (1987). Haloperidol deconoate: A preliminary review of its pharmacodynamic and pharmacokinetic properties and therapeutic use in psychosis. *Drugs, 33,* 31–49.

Berger, P. A. (1978). Medical treatment of mental illness. *Science, 200,* 974–981.

Berney, T. B., Kolvin, I., Bhate, S. R., Garside, R. F., Jeans, J., Kay, B. & Scarth, L. (1981). School phobia: A therapeutic trial with clomipramine and outcome. *British Journal of Psychiatry, 138,* 110–118.

Bianchine, J. R. (1985). Drugs for Parkinson's disease, spasticity, and acute muscle spasms. In A. F. Gilman, L. S. Goodman, T. W. Rall & F. Murad (Eds.), *The pharmacological basis of therapeutics* (pp. 473–490). New York: Macmillan.

Biederman, J., Baldessarini, R. J., Wright, V., Knee, D. & Harmatz, J. S. (1989). A double-blind placebo controlled study of desipramine in the treatment of ADD: I. Efficacy. *Journal of the American Academy of Child and Adolescent Psychiatry, 28,* 777–784.

Birch, N. J. (1980). Bone side-effects of lithium. In F. N. Johnson (Ed.), *Handbook of lithium therapy* (pp. 365–371). Lancaster, England: MTP Press.

Birhamer, B., Greenhill, L. L., Cooper, T. B., Fried, J. & Maminski, B. (1989). Sustained release methylphenidate: Pharmacokinetic studies in ADDH males. *Journal of the American Academy of Child and Adolescent Psychiatry, 28,* 768–772.

Blackwell, B. & Currah, J. (1973). The psychopharmacology of nocturnal enuresis. In I. Kalvin, R. C. MacKeith & S. R. Meadow (Eds.), *Bladder control and enuresis* (pp. 231–257). London: Heinemann.

Blaschke, T. G., Nies, A. S. & Mamelok, R. D. (1985). Principles of therapeutics. In

A. G. Gilman, L. S. Goodman, T. W. Rall & F. Murad (Eds.), *The pharmacological basis of therapeutics* (pp. 49–65). New York: Macmillan.

Borison, R. (1985, May). *The recognition and management of drug-induced movement disorders (reversible type).* Paper presented at the annual meeting of the American Psychiatric Association, Dallas, TX.

Bosco, J. & Robin, S. (1980). Hyperkinesis: Prevalence and treatment. In C. Whalen & B. Henker (Eds.), *Hyperactive children: The social ecology of identification and treatment* (pp. 173–187). New York: Academic Press.

Bossi, L. (1983). Fetal effects of anticonvulsants. In P. L. Morselli, C. E. Pippenger & J. E. Penry (Eds.), *Antiepilepsy drug therapy in pediatrics* (pp. 37–64). New York: Raven Press.

Bradley, C. (1937). The behavior of children receiving Benzedrine. *American Journal of Psychiatry, 94,* 577–585.

Bradley, C. (1950). Benzedrine and dexedrine in the treatment of children's behavior disorders. *Pediatrics, 5,* 24–37.

Bradley, C. & Bowen, M. (1941). Amphetamine (Benzedrine) therapy of children's behavior disorders. *American Journal of Orthopsychiatry, 11,* 92–103.

Braude, W. M., Barnes, T. R. E. & Gore, S. M. (1983). Clinical characteristics of akathisia: A systematic investigation of acute psychiatric inpatient admissions. *British Journal of Psychiatry, 143,* 139–150.

Briant, R. H. (1978). An introduction to clinical pharmacology. In J. S. Werry (Ed.), *Pediatric psychopharmacology: The use of behavior modifying drugs in children* (pp. 3–28). New York: Brunner/Mazel.

Brown, D., Winsberg, B. G., Bialer, I. & Press, M. (1973). Imipramine therapy and seizures: Three children treated for hyperactive behavior disorders. *American Journal of Psychiatry, 130,* 210–212.

Burns, D., Brady, J. P. & Kuruvilla, K. (1978). The acute effect of haloperidol and apomorphine on the severity of stuttering. *Biological Psychiatry, 13,* 255–264.

Cade, J. F. J. (1949). Lithium salts in the treatment of psychotic excitement. *Medical Journal of Australia, 36,* 349–352.

Campbell, M., Anderson, L. T., Deutsch, S. I. & Green, W. H. (1984c). Psychopharmacological treatment of children with the syndrome of autism. *Pediatric Annals, 13,* 309–316.

Campbell, M., Anderson, L. T., Meier, M., Cohen, I. L., Small, A. M., Samit, C. & Sachar, E. J. (1978). A comparison of haloperidol and behavior therapy and their interaction with autistic children. *Journal of the American Academy of Child Psychiatry, 17,* 640–655.

Campbell, M., Perry, R. & Green, W. H. (1984a). Use of lithium in children and adolescents. *Psychosomatics, 2,* 95–106.

Campbell, M., Small, A. M., Green, W. H., Jennings, S. J., Perry, R., Bennett, W. G. & Anderson, L. (1984b). Behavioral efficacy of haloperidol and lithium carbonate: A comparison in hospitalized aggressive children with conduct disorder. *Archives of General Psychiatry, 120,* 650–656.

Campbell, S. B., Endman, M. W. & Bernfeld, G. (1977). A three-year follow-up of hyperactive preschoolers into elementary school. *Journal of Child Psychology and Psychiatry, 18,* 239–249.

Cantwell, D. P. & Carlson, G. A. (1978). Stimulants. In J. S. Werry (Ed.), *Pediatric psychopharmacology: The use of behavior modifying drugs with children* (pp. 171–207). New York: Brunner/Mazel.

Carlson, G. A. (1983). Bipolar affective disorders in childhood and adolescence. In D. P. Cantwell & G. A. Carlson (Eds.), *Affective disorders in childhood and adolescence: An update* (pp. 61–83). New York: Spectrum.

Carlson, G. A. (1986). Classification issues of bipolar disorder in childhood. *Psychiatric Development, 6,* 273–285.

Carlson, G. A. & Cantwell, D. P. (1980). Unmasking masked depression in children and adolescents. *American Journal of Psychiatry, 137,* 445–449.

Charles, L. & Schain, R. (1981). A four-year follow-up study of the effects of methylphenidate on the behavior and academic achievement of hyperactive children. *Journal of Abnormal Child Psychology, 9,* 494–505.

Chatoor, I., Wells, K. C., Conners, C. K., Seidel, W. T. & Shaw, D. (1983). The effects of nocturnally administered stimulant medication on EEG sleep and behavior in hyperactive children. *Journal of the American Academy of Child Psychiatry, 22,* 337–342.

Chouinard, G., Montigny, C. D. & Annable, L. (1979). Tardive dyskinesia and antiparkinsonian medication. *American Journal of Psychiatry, 136,* 228–229.

Clark, W. G. & del Guidice, J. (1978). *Principles of psychopharmacology.* New York: Academic Press.

Cohen, W. J. & Cohen, N. H. (1974). Lithium carbonate, haloperidol, and irreversible brain damage. *Journal of the American Medical Association, 230,* 1283–1287.

Cole, J. O. (1988). Where are those new antidepressants we were promised? *Archives of General Psychiatry, 45,* 193–194.

Commission on Classification and Terminology of the International League Against Epilepsy. Proposal for revised clinical and electroencephalographic classification of epileptic seizures. *Epilepsia, 22,* 489–491.

Conners, C. K. (1969). A teacher rating scale for use in drug studies with children. *American Journal of Psychiatry, 126,* 884–888.

Conners, C. K. (1973). Rating scales for use in drug studies with children. *Psychopharmacology Bulletin* (special issue, Pharmacotherapy of children), 24–84.

Conners, C. K. (1980). *Food additives and hyperactive children.* New York: Plenum Press.

Conners, C. K. & Werry, J. S. (1979). Psychopharmacology. In H. Quay & J. S. Werry (Eds.), *Psychopathological disorders of childhood* (pp. 416–478). New York: John Wiley & Sons.

Conners, C. K., Taylor, E., Meo, G., Jurtz, M. A. & Fournier, M. (1972). Magnesium pemoline and dextroamphetamine: A controlled study in children with minimum brain dysfunction. *Psychopharmacologia, 26,* 321–336.

Connor, J. D. (1984). Antipsychotic and antianxiety and drugs. In A. Goth (Ed.), *Medical pharmcology* (pp. 251–268). St. Louis: Mosby.

Coons, D. J., Hillman, F. J. & Marshall, R. W. (1982). Treatment of neuroleptic malignant syndrome with dantrolene sodium: A case report. *American Journal of Psychiatry, 139,* 944–945.

Cooper, A. F. & Fowlie, H. C. (1973). Control of gross self-mutilation with lithium carbonate. *British Journal of Psychiatry, 122,* 370–371.

Cott, A. (1972). Megavitamins: The orthomolecular approach to behavioral disorders and learning disabilities. *Academic Therapy, 7,* 245–258.

Cramer, J. A., Smith, D. B., Mattson, R. H., Excueta, A. V. D., Cellins, J. F., & the VA Cooperative Study Group. (1983). A method of quantification for the evaluation of antiepileptic drug therapy. *Neurology, 33* (Suppl. 1), 26–27.

Crane, G. E. (1959). Iproniazid (Marsilid) phosphate, a therapeutic agent for mental disorders and debilitating disease. *Psychiatric Research Reports, 8,* 142–152.

Crook, T. H., Kupfer, D. J., Hoch, C. C. & Reynolds, C. F. (1987). Treatment of sleep disorders in the elderly. In H. Y. Meltzer (Ed.), *Psychopharmacology: The third generation of progress* (pp. 1159–1166). New York: Raven Press.

Davis, J. M. (1975). Overview: Maintenance therapy in schizophrenia. I. Schizophrenia. *American Journal of Psychiatry, 132,* 1237–1265.

Davis, J. M. (1976). Comparative doses and costs of neuroleptic drugs. *Archives of General Psychiatry, 33*, 858–861.

DeLong, G. R. (1978). Lithium carbonate treatment of select behavior disorders in children suggesting manic-depressive illness. *Journal of Pediatrics, 93*, 689–694.

DeLong, G. R. & Aldershof, A. L. (1987). Long-term experience with lithium treatment in childhood: Correlation with clinical diagnosis. *Journal of the American Academy of Child and Adolescent Psychiatry, 26*, 389–394.

DeVito, D. C. (1983). Myoclonic seizures. In P. L. Morselli, C. E. Pippenger & J. E. Penry (Eds.), *Antiepilepsy drug therapy in pediatrics* (pp. 137–143). New York: Raven Press.

Dimijian, G. G. (1984). Contemporary drug abuse. In A. Goth (Ed.), *Medical pharmacology* (pp. 336–365). St. Louis: Mosby.

Dreifuss, F. E. (1982). Ethosuximide toxicity. In D. M. Woodbury, J. K. Penry & C. E. Pippenger (Eds.), *Antiepileptic drugs* (pp. 647–654). New York: Raven Press.

Dunner, D. L., Vijayalasky, P. & Fieve, R. R. (1977). Rapid cycling manic depressive patients. *Comprehensive Psychiatry, 18*, 561–565.

Durand, V. M. (1982). A behavioral/pharmacological intervention for the treatment of severe self-injurious behavior. *Journal of Autism and Developmental Disorders, 12*, 243–251.

Durand, V. M. (1986). Self-injurious behavior as intentional communication. In K. D. Gadow (Ed.), *Advances in learning and behavioral disabilities* (Vol. 5., pp. 141–155). Greenwich, CT: JAI Press.

Durand, V. M. (1987). Look homeward angel: A call to return to our functional roots. *The Behavior Analyst, 10*, 299–302.

Dykman, R. A., McGrew, J. & Ackerman, P. T. (1974). A double-blind clinical study of pemoline in MBD children: Comments on the psychological test result. In C. K. Conners (Ed.), *Clinical use of stimulant drugs in children* (pp. 123–176). New York: Elsevier.

Eichlseder, W. (1985). Ten years of experience with 1,000 hyperactive children in a private practice. *Pediatrics, 76*, 176–184.

Elkins, R., Rapoport, J. L. & Lipsky, A. (1980). Obsessive-compulsive disorder of childhood and adolescence: A neurobiological viewpoint. *Journal of the American Academy of Child Psychiatry, 19*, 511–524.

Engelhardt, D. M. (1974). *Withdrawal Emergent Symptoms (WES) Checklist.* Unpublished manuscript.

Epilepsy Foundation of America. (1975). *Basic statistics on the epilepsies.* Philadelphia: F. A. Davis.

Farber, J. M. (1987). Psychopharmacology of self-injurious behavior in the mentally retarded. *Journal of the American Academy of Child and Adolescent Psychiatry, 26*, 296–302.

Fazen, L. E., Lovejoy, F. H. & Crone, R. K. (1986). Acute poisoning in a children's hospital: A 2-year experience. *Pediatrics, 77*, 144–151.

Fielding, L. T., Murphy, R. J., Reagan, M. W. & Peterson, T. L. (1980). An assessment program to reduce drug use with the mentally retarded. *Hospital and Community Psychiatry, 31*, 771–773.

Feingold, B. F. (1974). *Why your child is hyperactive.* New York: Random House.

Fisher, W., Kerbeshian, J. & Burd, L. (1986). A treatable language disorder: Pharmacological treatment of pervasive developmental disorder. *Developmental and Behavioral Pediatrics, 7*, 73–76.

Flament, M. F., Rapoport, J. L., Berg, C. J., Sceery, W., Kilts, L., Mellstrom, B. & Linnoila, M. (1985). Clomipramine treatment of childhood obsessive-compulsive disorders. *Archives of General Psychiatry, 42*, 977–983.

Franz, D. N. (1985). Central nervous system stimulants. In A. G. Gilman, L. S. Goodman, T. W. Rall & F. Murad (Eds.), *The pharmacological basis of therapeutics* (pp. 582–589). New York: Macmillan.

Freeman, J., Holden, K. & Pillas, D. (1977). *Approaches to the improved care of institutionalized epileptic persons*. Washington, DC: U.S. Government Printing Office.

Freeman, L. N., Poznanski, E. O., Grossman, J. A., Buchsbaum, Y. Y. & Banegas, M. E. (1985). Psychotic and depressed children: A new entity. *Journal of the American Academy of Child Psychiatry, 24,* 95–102.

Friedel, R. O. (1984). An overview of neuroleptic plasma levels: Pharmacokinetics and assay methodology. *Journal of Clinical Psychiatry Monograph, 2,* 7–12.

Fromm, G. H., Wessel, H. B., Glass, J. D., Alvin, J. D. & van Horn, G. (1978). Imipramine in absence and myoclonic-astatic seizures. *Neurology, 28,* 953–957.

Gadow, K. D. (1981). Prevalence of drug treatment for hyperactivity and other childhood behavior disorders. In K. D. Gadow & J. Loney (Eds.), *Psychosocial aspects of drug treatment for hyperactivity* (pp. 13–76). Boulder, CO: Westview.

Gadow, K. D. (1985). Relative efficacy of pharmacological, behavioral, and combination treatments for enhancing academic performance. *Clinical Psychology Review, 5,* 513–533.

Gadow, K. D. (1986a). *Children on medication: Vol. I. Hyperactivity, learning disabilities, and mental retardation*. San Diego: College-Hill Press.

Gadow, K. D. (1986b). *Children on medication: Vol. II. Epilepsy, emotional disturbance, and adolescent disorders*. San Diego: College-Hill Press.

Gadow, K. D. & Kalachnik, J. (1981). Prevalence and pattern of drug treatment for behavior and seizure disorders of TMR students. *American Journal of Mental Deficiency, 85,* 588–595.

Gadow, K. D., Nolan, E. E., Sverd, J., Sprafkin, J., & Paolicelli, L. (in press). Methylphenidate in aggressive-hyperactive boys: I. Effects on peer aggression in public school settings. *Journal of the American Academy of Child and Adolescent Psychiatry.*

Gadow, K. D. & Poling, A. (1986). *Methodological issues in human psychopharmacology (Advances in learning and behavioral disabilities, Suppl. 1)*. Greenwich, CT: JAI Press.

Gadow, K. D. & Poling, A. (1988). *Pharmacotherapy in mental retardation*. San Diego: College-Hill Press.

Gadow, K. D., White, L. & Ferguson, D. G. (1986a). Placebo controls and double-blind conditions: Experimenter bias, conditioned placebo response, and drug-psychotherapy comparisons. In K. D. Gadow & A. Poling (Eds.), *Methodological issues in human psychopharmacology (Advances in learning and behavioral disabilities, Suppl. 1)* (pp. 85–114). Greenwich, CT: JAI Press.

Gadow, K. D., White, L. & Ferguson, D. G. (1986b). Placebo controls and double-blind conditions: Placebo theory in experimental design. In K. D. Gadow & A. Poling (Eds.), *Methodological issues in human psychopharmacology (Advances in learning and behavioral disabilities, Suppl. 1)* (pp. 41–84). Greenwich, CT: JAI Press.

Gardos, G., Cole, J. O., Salomon, M. & Schniebolk, S. (1987). Clinical forms of severe tardive dyskinesia. *American Journal of Psychiatry, 144,* 895–902.

Gardos, G., Perenyi, A., Cole, J. O., Samu, I. & Kallos, M. (1983). Tardive dyskinesia: Changes after three years. *Journal of Clinical Psychopharmacology, 3,* 315–318.

Gastaut, H. (1970). Clinical and electroencephalographical classification of epileptic seizures. *Epilepsia, 11,* 102–113.

Gattozzi, A. A. (1970). *Lithium in the treatment of mood disorders*. Washington, DC: U.S. Government Printing Office.

Geller, B., Chestnut, E. C., Miller, M. D., Price, D. T. & Yates, E. (1985). Preliminary data on DSM III associated features of major depressive disorder in children and adolescents. *American Journal of Psychiatry, 142,* 643–644.

Gerson, S. C., Plotkin, D. A. & Jarvik, L. F. (1988). Antidepressant drug studies, 1964 to 1986: Empirical evidence for aging patients. *Journal of Clinical Psychopharmacology, 8,* 311–322.

Gibbs, E. L., Gibbs, T. J., Gibbs, R. A., Gibbs, E. A., Dikmen, S. & Hermann, B. P. (1982). Antiepilepsy drugs. In S. E. Breuning & A. Poling (Eds.), *Drugs and mental retardation* (pp. 268–329). Springfield, IL: Charles C Thomas.

Gitlin, M. J., Cochran, S. D. & Jamison, K. R. (1989). Maintenance lithium treatment: Side effects and compliance. *Journal of Clinical Psychiatry, 50*, 127–131.

Gittelman-Klein, R. (1975a). Introduction: Recent advances in child psychopharmacology. *International Journal of Mental Health, 4*, 3–10.

Gittelman-Klein, R. (1975b). Pharmacotherapy and management of pathological separation anxiety. *International Journal of Mental Health, 4*, 255–271.

Gittelman-Klein, R. & Klein, D. F. (1971). Controlled imipramine treatment of school phobia. *Archives of General Psychiatry, 25*, 204–207.

Gittelman-Klein, R., Klein, D. G., Katz, S., Saraf, K. & Pollack, E. (1976). Comparative effects of methylphenidate and thioridazine in hyperkinetic children. *Archives of General Psychiatry, 33*, 1217–1231.

Gofman, H. (1972–1973). Interval and final rating sheets on side-effects. *Psychopharmacology Bulletin* (Special Issue), *8–9*, 182–187.

Goodyer, I. M. (1985). Epileptic and pseudoseizures in childhood and adolescence. *Journal of the American Academy of Child Psychiatry, 24*, 3–9.

Goth, A. (1985). *Medical pharmacology*, St. Louis: Mosby.

Gowdey, C. W., Coleman, L. M. & Crawford, E. M. (1985). Ocular changes and phenothiazine derivatives in long-term residents of a mental retardation center. *Psychiatric Journal of the University of Ottawa, 10*, 248–253.

Greaves, G. B. (1980). Psychosocial aspects of amphetamine and related substance abuse. In J. Caldwell (Ed.), *Amphetamines and related stimulants: Chemical, biological, clinical and sociological aspects* (pp. 175–192). Boca Raton, FL: CRC.

Green, W. H., Campbell, M., Hardesty, A. S., Grega, D. M., Padron-Gayol, M., Shell, J. & Erlenmeyer-Kimling, L. (1984). A comparison of schizophrenic and autistic children. *Journal of the American Academy of Child Psychiatry, 23*, 399–409.

Greenblat, D. J., Shader, R. I. & Abernathy, D. R. (1978). Current status of benzodiazepines. *New England Journal of Medicine, 309*, 410–416.

Greiner, T. (1958). Problems of methodology in research with drugs. *American Journal of Mental Deficiency, 64*, 346–352.

Griffin, J. C., Williams, D. E., Stark, M. T., Altmeyer, B. K. & Mason, M. (1986). Self-injurious behavior: A state-wide prevalence survey of the extent and circumstances. *Applied Research in Mental Retardation, 7*, 105–116.

Hamilton, M. (1967). Development of a rating scale for primary depressive illness. *British Journal of School and Clinical Psychology, 6*, 278–296.

Harvey, S. C. (1985). Sedatives and hypnotics. In A. F. Gilman, L. S. Goodman, T. W. Rall & F. Murad (Eds.), *The pharmacological basis of therapeutics* (pp. 339–371). New York: Macmillan.

Haslam, R. H. A., Dalby, J. T. & Rademaker, A. W. (1984). Effects of megavitamin therapy on children with attention deficit disorders. *Pediatrics, 74*, 103–111.

Hauser, W. A. (1978). Epidemiology of epilepsy. *Advances in Neurology, 19*, 313–339.

Haynes, R. B., Taylor, D. W. & Sackett, D. L. (1979). *Compliance in health care.* Baltimore: Johns Hopkins Press.

Hersen, M. (1986). Introduction. In M. Hersen (Ed.), *Pharmacological and behavioral treatment: An integrative approach* (pp. 5–14). New York: John Wiley & Sons.

Hersen, M. & Barlow, D. J. (1976). *Single case experimental designs.* Elmsford, NY: Pergamon Press.

Hogarty, G. E. & Ulrich, R. F. (1977). Temporal effects of drug and placebo in delaying response in schizophrenic out-patients. *Archives of General Psychiatry, 34*, 297–301.

Hooshmand, H. (1978). A look at the EEG report. *Clinical EEG, 9,* 118–123.

Howell, L. (1978). Epilepsy. In R. M. Goldenson, J. R. Dunham & C. S. Dunham (Eds.), *Disability and rehabilitation handbook* (pp. 381–388). New York: McGraw-Hill.

Iwata, B. A. & Bailey, J. S. (1974). Reward versus cost token systems: An analysis of the effects on students and teachers. *Journal of Applied Behavior Analysis, 7,* 567–576.

Jaffee, J. H. (1985). Drug addiction and drug abuse. In A. G. Gilman, L. S. Goodman, T. W. Rall & F. Murad (Eds.), *The pharmacological basis of therapeutics* (pp. 532–581). New York: Macmillan.

James, D. H. (1986). Neuroleptics and epilepsy in mentally handicapped patients. *Journal of Mental Deficiency Research, 30,* 185–189.

Jann, M. W., Ereshefsky, L., Saklad, S. R., Seidel, D. R., Davis, C. M., Burch, N. R. & Bowden, C. L. (1985). Effects of carbamazepine on plasma haloperidol levels. *Journal of Clinical Psychopharmacology, 5,* 106–109.

Jeavons, P. M. (1982). Valproate toxicity. In D. M. Woodbury, J. K. Penry & C. E. Pippenger (Eds.), *Antiepileptic drugs* (pp. 601–610). New York: Raven Press.

Johnson, D. A. W. (1976). The expectation of outcome from maintenance therapy in chronic schizophrenic patients. *British Journal of Psychiatry, 128,* 246–250.

Johnson, D. A. W. (1984). Observations on the use of long-acting depot neuroleptic injections in the maintenance therapy of schizophrenia. *Journal of Clinical Psychiatry, 45,* 13–21.

Judd, L. L., Squire, L. R., Butters, W., Salmon, D. P. & Paller, K. A. (1987). Effects of psychotropic drugs on cognition and memory in normal humans and animals. In H. Y. Meltzer (Ed.), *Psychopharmacology: The third generation of progress* (pp. 1467–1475). New York: Raven Press.

Julien, R. M. (1988). *A primer of drug action.* San Francisco: Freeman.

Kalachnik, J. E. (1985). *Monitoring of side-effects scale (MOSES).* Unpublished manuscript.

Kalachnik, J. E. (1988). Medication monitoring procedures. In K. D. Gadow & A. Poling, *Pharmacotherapy and mental retardation* (pp. 231–268). San Diego: College-Hill Press.

Kales, A. & Kales, J. D. (1983). Sleep laboratory studies of hypnotic drugs: Efficacy and withdrawal effects. *Journal of Clinical Psychopharmacology, 3,* 140.

Kane, J. M. (1983). Problems of compliance in the outpatient treatment of schizophrenia. *Journal of Clinical Psychiatry, 44,* 3–6.

Kashani, J. H. & Simonds, J. F. (1979). The incidence of depression in children. *American Journal of Psychiatry, 136,* 1203–1205.

Katz, S., Saraf, K., Gittelman-Klein, R. & Klein, D. F. (1975). Clinical pharmacological management of hyperkinetic children. *International Journal of Mental Health, 4,* 157–181.

Kazdin, A. E. (1982). *Single-case research designs.* New York: Oxford.

Kinsbourne, M. & Swanson, J. M. (1979). Models of hyperactivity. In R. L. Trites (Ed.), *Hyperactivity in children* (pp. 365–436). Baltimore: University Park Press.

Klein, D. F. (1981). Anxiety reconceptualized. In D. F. Klein & J. G. Rabkin (Eds.), *Anxiety: New research and current concepts* (pp. 138–213). New York: Raven Press.

Klein, D. F. & Fink, M. (1962). Psychiatric reaction patterns to imipramine. *American Journal of Psychiatry, 119,* 432–438.

Klein, D. F., Gittelman-Klein, R., Quitkin, F. & Rifkin, A. (1980). *Diagnosis and drug treatment of psychiatric disorders: Adults and children.* Baltimore: Williams & Wilkins.

Kline, N. S. (1958). Clinical experience with iproniazid (Marsilid). *Journal of Clinical and Experimental Psychopathology, 19,* 72–78.

Knopp, W., Arnold, L. E., Andras, R. L. & Smeltzer, D. J. (1973). Predicting amphetamine response in hyperkinetic children by electric pupillography. *Pharmakopsychiatrie Neuropsychopharmakologie, 6,* 158–166.

Kolvin, I., Berney, T. P., & Bhate, S. R. (1984). Classification and diagnosis of depression in school phobia. *British Journal of Psychiatry, 145,* 347–357.

Kolvin, I., Taunch, J., Currah, J., Garside, R. F., Nolan, J. & Shaw, W. B. (1972). Enuresis: A descriptive analysis and a controlled trial. *Developmental Medicine and Child Neurology, 14,* 715–726.

Kovacs, M., Feinberg, T. L., Crouse-Novak, M. A., Paulauskas, S. L. & Finkelstein, R. (1984). Depressive disorders in childhood: I. A longitudinal prospective study of characteristics and recovery. *Archives of General Psychiatry, 41,* 229–237.

Kramer, A. D., & Feiguine, R. J. (1981). Clinical effects of amitriptyline in adolescent depression: A pilot study. *Journal of the American Academy of Child Psychiatry, 20,* 636–644.

Kramer, M. S., Vogel, W. H., Di Johnson, C., Dewey, D. A., Sheves, P., Cavicchia, S., Little, P., Schmidt, R. & Kimes, I. (1989). Antidepressants in "depressed" psychiatric inpatients. *Archives of General Psychiatry, 46,* 922–928.

Kuhn, R. (1958). The treatment of depressive states with G22355 (imipramine hydrochloride). *American Journal of Psychiatry, 115,* 459–464.

Kumar, B. B. (1979). An unusual case of akathisia. *American Journal of Psychiatry, 136,* 1083.

Kupfer, D. J., Carpenter, L. L. & Frank, E. (1988). Possible role of antidepressants in precipitating mania and hypomania in recurrent depression. *American Journal of Psychiatry, 145,* 804–808.

Lader, M. (1989). Clinical pharmacology of antipsychotic drugs. *Journal of International Medical Research, 17,* 1–16.

Lansky, M. R. & Selzer, J. (1984). Priapism associated with trazodone therapy: Case report. *Journal of Clinical Psychiatry, 45,* 232–233.

Lewis, J. A. & Lewis, B. S. (1977). Deanol in minimal brain dysfunction. *Diseases of the Nervous System, 38,* 21–24.

Lewis, J. L. & Winokur, G. (1982). The induction of mania. *Archives of General Psychiatry, 39,* 303–306.

Lickey, M. E. & Gordon, B. (1983). *Drugs for mental illness.* San Francisco: Freeman.

Lipinski, J. F., Zubenko, G. S., Cohen, B. M. & Barreira, P. J. (1984). Propranolol in the treatment of neuroleptic-induced akathisia. *American Journal of Psychiatry, 141,* 412–415.

Lipton, M. A., DiMascio, A. & Killam, K. F. (1978). *Psychopharmacology: A generation of progress.* New York: Raven Press.

Livingston, S. (1972). *Comprehensive management of epilepsy in infancy.* Springfield, IL: Charles C Thomas.

Livingston, S. (1978). Medical treatment of epilepsy: Part II. *Southern Medical Journal, 71,* 298–310.

Longo, V. G. (1972). *Neuropharmacology and behavior.* San Francisco: Freeman.

Lydiard, R. B. & Gelenberg, A. J. (1982). Hazards and adverse effects of lithium. *Annual Review of Medicine, 33,* 327–344.

Lydiard, R. B., Roy-Byrne, P. P. & Ballenger, J. C. (1988). Recent advances in the psychopharmacological treatment of anxiety disorders. *Hospital and Community Psychiatry, 39,* 1157–1165.

MacLean, R. E. G. (1960). Imipramine hydrochloride and enuresis. *American Journal of Psychiatry, 117,* 551.

Marder, S. R., Hawes, E. M. & Van Patten, T. (1986). Fluphenazine plasma levels in patients receiving low and conventional doses of fluphenazine decanoate. *Psychopharmacology, 88,* 480–483.

Marholin, D., Touchette, P. E. & Stewart, R. M. (1979). Withdrawal of chronic chlorpromazine medication: An experimental analysis. *Journal of Applied Behavior Analysis, 12,* 150–171.

Martin, J. E. & Agran, M. (1985). Psychotropic and anticonvulsant drug use by mentally retarded adults across community residential and vocational placements. *Applied Research in Mental Retardation, 6,* 33–49.

Mash, E. J. & Dalby, J. T. (1979). Behavioral interventions for hyperactivity. In R. L. Trites (Ed.), *Hyperactivity in children* (pp. 137–173). Baltimore: University Park Press.

May, P. R. A. (1968). *Treatment of schizophrenia: A comparative study of five treatment methods.* New York: Science House.

McEvoy, G. K. (1988). *American hospital formulary service drug information 89.* New York: American Society of Hospital Pharmacists.

McEvoy, J. P. (1983). The clinical use of anticholinergic drugs as treatment for extrapyramidal side effects of neuroleptic drugs. *Journal of Clinical Psychopharmacology, 3,* 288–302.

McEvoy, J. P., McCue, M., Spring, B., Mohs, R. C., Lavori, P. W. & Farr, R. M. (1987). Effects of amantadine and trihexyphenidyl on memory in elderly normal volunteers. *American Journal of Psychiatry, 144,* 573–577.

Meadow, R. & Berg, I. (1982). Controlled trial of imipramine in diurnal enuresis. *Archives of Disease in Childhood, 57,* 714–716.

Medical Letters. (1976). *18,* 18–19.

Menolascino, F. J., Ruedrich, S. L., Golden, C. J. & Wilson, J. E. (1985). Diagnosis and pharmacotherapy of schizophrenia in the retarded. *Psychopharmacology Bulletin, 21,* 316–322.

Moore, D. J. & Klonoff, E. A. (1986). Assessment of compliance: A systems perspective. In K. D. Gadow & A. Poling (Eds.), *Methodological issues in human psychopharmacology (Advances in learning and behavioral disabilities, Suppl. 1)* (pp. 223–246). Greenwich, CT: JAI Press.

Morris, J. B. & Beck, A. T. (1974). The efficacy of antidepressant drugs. *Archives of General Psychiatry, 30,* 667–674.

Morselli, P. L., Pippenger, C. E. & Penry, J. E. (1983). *Antiepilepsy drug therapy in pediatrics.* New York: Raven Press.

Mueller, P. S., Vester, J. W. & Fermaglich, J. (1983). Neuroleptic malignant syndrome: Successful treatment with bromocriptine. *Journal of the American Medical Association, 249,* 386–388.

Munetz, M. R. & Cornes, C. L. (1983). Distinguishing akathisia and tardive dyskinesia: A review of the literature. *Journal of Clinical Psychopharmacology, 3,* 343–350.

National Institutes of Mental Health, Psychopharmacology Service Center. (1964). Phenothiazine in acute schizophrenia. *Archives of General Psychiatry, 10,* 246–261.

National Institutes of Mental Health. (1985a). DOTES (Dosage Record and Treatment Emergent Symptom Scale). *Psychopharmacology Bulletin, 20,* 1067–1068.

National Institutes of Mental Health. (1985b). STRESS (Subjective Treatment Emergent Symptoms Scale). *Psychopharmacology Bulletin, 20,* 1073–1075.

National Institutes of Mental Health. (1986). Systematic Assessment for Treatment Emergent Events (SAFTEE). *Psychopharmacology Bulletin, 22,* 347–381.

National Institute on Drug Abuse. (1978). *Behavioral tolerance: Research and treatment implications.* Washington, DC: U.S. Government Printing Office.

Noyes, R., Garvey, M. J., Cook, B. L. & Samuelson, L. (1989). Problems with tricyclic antidepressant use in patients with panic disorder or agoraphobia: Results of a naturalistic followup study. *Journal of Clinical Psychiatry, 50,* 163–169.

O'Leary, K. D. (1980). Pills or skills for hyperactive children. *Journal of of Applied Behavior Analysis, 13,* 191–204.

Page, T. J. & Iwata, B. A. (1986). Interobserver agreement: History, theory, and current methods. In A. Poling & R. W. Fuqua (Eds.), *Research methods in applied behavior analysis* (pp. 99–126). New York: Plenum Press.

Pasnau, P. O. (1984). Clinical presentations of panic and anxiety. *Psychosomatics, 25,* 4–9.

Paul, G. L. (1967). Strategy of outcome research in psychotherapy. *Journal of Consulting Psychology, 31,* 104–118.

Pelham, W. E. (1983). The effects of psychostimulants on academic achievement in hyperactive and learning-disabled children. *Thalamus, 3,* 1–47.

Pelham, W. E. & Bender, M. E. (1982). Peer relations in children with hyperactivity/attention deficit disorder. In K. D. Gadow & I. Bailer (Eds.), *Advances in learning and behavioral disabilities* (Vol. 1, pp. 365–436). Greenwich, CT: JAI Press.

Pelham, W. E. & Murphy, A. (1986). Attention deficit and conduct disorders. In M. Hersen (Ed.), *Pharmacological and behavioral treatment: An integrative approach* (pp. 108–148). New York: John Wiley & Sons.

Pelham, W. E., Bender, M. E., Caddell, J., Booth, S. & Moorer, S. H. (1985). Methylphenidate and children with attention deficit and conduct disorders: Dose effects on classroom academic and social behavior. *Archives of General Psychiatry, 42,* 948–952.

Perry, R., Campbell, M., Grega, D. M. & Anderson, L. (1984). Saliva lithium level in children: Their use in monitoring serum lithium levels and lithium side effects. *Journal of Clinical Psychopharmacology, 4,* 199–202.

Pietsch, S. (1977). *The person with epilepsy: Life style, needs, expectations.* Chicago: National Epilepsy League.

Pliszka, S. R. (1987). Tricyclic antidepressants in the treatment of children with attention deficit disorder. *Journal of of the American Academy of Child and Adolescent Psychiatry, 26,* 127–132.

Poling, A (1986). *A primer of human behavioral pharmacology.* New York: Plenum Press.

Pool, D., Bloom, W., Mielke, D. H., Roniger, J. J. & Gallant, D. M. (1976). A controlled evaluation of loxitane in seventy-five schizophrenic patients. *Current Therapeutic Research, 19,* 99–104.

Pope, H. G., Hudson, J. I., Jonas, J. M., Yurgelun-Todd, D. (1983). Bulimia treated with imipramine: A placebo-controlled, double-blind study. *American Journal of Psychiatry, 140,* 554–558.

Pope, H. G., Keck, P. E. & McElroy, S. L. (1986). Frequency of neuroleptic malignant syndrome in a large psychiatric hospital. *American Journal of Psychiatry, 143,* 1227–1233.

Preskorn, S. H. (1989). Tricyclic antidepressants: The whys and hows of therapeutic drug monitoring. *Journal of Clinical Psychiatry, 50,* 34–42.

Prinz, R. J. (1985). Diet-behavior research with children: Methodological and substantive issues. In K. D. Gadow (Ed.), *Advances in learning and behavioral disabilities* (Vol. 4, pp. 181–199). Greenwich, CT: JAI Press.

Puig-Antich, J. (1982). Major depression and conduct disorder in prepuberty. *Journal of the American Academy of Child Psychiatry, 21,* 118–128.

Puig-Antich, J., Perel, J. M., Lupatkin, W., Chambers, W. J., Tabrinzi, M. A., King, J., Goetz, R., Davies, M. & Stiller, R. L. (1987). Imipramine in prepubertal major depressive disorders. *Archives of General Psychiatry, 44,* 81–89.

Quality Assurance Project. (1984). Treatment outlines for the management of schizophrenia. *Australian and New Zealand Journal of Psychiatry, 18,* 19–38.

Quinn, P. O. & Rapoport, J. L. (1975). One-year follow-up of hyperactive boys treated with imipramine or methylphenidate. *American Journal of Psychiatry, 132,* 241–245.

Quinn, P. T. & Peachey, E. C. (1973). Haloperidol for the treatment of stutterers. *British Journal of Psychiatry, 123,* 247–255.

Rall, T. W. & Schliefer, L. S. (1985). Drugs effective in the therapy of the epilepsies. In A. G. Gilman, L. S. Goodman, T. W. Rall & F. Murad (Eds.), *The pharmacological basis of therapeutics* (pp. 446–472). New York: Macmillan.

Rapoport, J. L., Buschbaum, M., Weingartner, H., Zahn, T. P. & Ludlow, C. (1980). Dextroamphetamine: Cognitive and behavioral effects in normal prepubertal boys. *Science, 199,* 560–563.

Rapoport, J. L., Buschbaum, M., Zahn, T. P., Weingartner, M., Ludlow, C. & Mikkelsen, E. J. (1978). Dextroamphetamine: Cognitive and behavioral effects in normal and hyperactive boys and normal men. *Archives of General Psychiatry, 37,* 933–943.

Rapoport, J. L., Quinn, P. O., Bradbard, G., Riddle, K. D. & Brooks, E. (1974). Imipramine and methylphenidate treatments of hyperactive boys. *Archives of General Psychiatry, 30,* 789–793.

Rapport, M. D., Murphy, H. A. & Bailey, J. S. (1982). Ritalin vs. response cost in the control of hyperactive children: A within-subject comparison. *Journal of Applied Behavior Analysis, 15,* 205–216.

Rapport, M. D., Stoner, G., DuPaul, G. J., Birmingham, B. K. & Tucker, S. (1985). Methylphenidate in hyperactive children: Differential effects of dose on academic, learning, and social behavior. *Journal of Abnormal Child Psychology, 13,* 227–244.

Ray, O. & Ksir, C. (1987). *Drugs, society, and human behavior.* St. Louis: Mosby.

Realmuto, G. M., Erickson, W. D., Yellin, A. M., Hopwood, J. H. & Greenberg, L. M. (1984). Clinical comparison of thiothixene and thioridazine in schizophrenic adolescents. *American Journal of Psychiatry, 141,* 440–442.

Reynolds, E. H. & Shorvon, S. D. (1981). Monotherapy or polytherapy for epilepsy? *Epilepsia, 22,* 1–20.

Riddle, D. & Rapoport, J. L. (1976). A 2-year follow up of 72 hyperactive boys. *Journal of Nervous and Mental Disease, 162,* 126–134.

Rifkin, A., Quitkin, F., Carillo, C., Blumberg, A. G. & Klein, D. F. (1972). Lithium carbonate in emotionally unstable character disorder. *Archives of General Psychiatry, 27,* 519–523.

Ritchie, J. M. (1985). The aliphatic alcohols. In A. F. Gilman, L. S. Goodman, T. W. Rall & F. Murad (Eds.), *The pharmacological basis of therapeutics* (pp. 372–386). New York: Macmillan.

Robinson, D. S. & Barker, E. (1976). Tricyclic antidepressant cardiotoxicity. *Journal of the American Medical Association, 236,* 2089–2090.

Romanczyk, R. G. (1986). Self-injurious behavior: Conceptualization, assessment, and treatment. In K. D. Gadow (Ed.), *Advances in learning and behavioral disabilities* (Vol. 5, pp. 29–56). Greenwich, CT: JAI Press.

Rosebush, P. & Stewart, T. (1989). A prospective analysis of 24 episodes of neuroleptic malignant syndrome. *American Journal of Psychiatry, 146,* 717–725.

Rosenbaum, J. F. (1982). The drug treatment of anxiety. *New England Journal of Medicine, 306,* 401–404.

Ross, D. A. & Ross, S. A. (1982). *Hyperactivity: Current issues, research, and theory.* New York: John Wiley & Sons.

Rotblatt, M. D. (1982). Antidepressants and seizures. *Drug Intelligence and Clinical Pharmacy, 16,* 749–750.

Ryan, N. D. & Puig-Antich, J. (1987). Pharmacological treatment of adolescent psychiatric disorders. *Journal of Adolescent Health Care, 8,* 137–142.

Ryan, N. D., Puig-Antich, J., Cooper, T. B., Rabinovich, H., Ambrosini, P., Fried, J., Davies, M., Torres, D., & Suckow, R. F. (1987). Relative safety of single versus divided dose imipramine in adolescent major depression. *Journal of the American Academy of Child and Adolescent Psychiatry, 26,* 400–406.

Ryan, N. D., Meyer, V., Dachille, S., Mazzie, D. & Puig-Antich, J. (1988a). Lithium antidepressant augmentation of TCA-refractory depression in adolescents. *Journal of the American Academy of Child and Adolescent Psychiatry, 27,* 371–376.

Ryan, N. D., Puig-Antich, J., Cooper, T. B., Rabinovich, H., Ambrosini, P. J., Davies,

M., King, J., Torres, D. & Fried, J. (1986). Imipramine in adolescent major depression: Plasma level and clinical response. *Acta Psychiatrica Scandinavica, 73,* 275–288.

Ryan, N. D., Puig-Antich, J., Rabinovich, H., Fried, J., Ambrosini, P., Meyer, V., Torres, D., Dachille, S. & Mazzie, D. (1988b). MAOIs in adolescent major depression unresponsive to tricyclic antidepressants. *Journal of the American Academy of Child and Adolescent Psychiatry, 27,* 755–758.

Safer, D. J. & Krager, J. M. (1984). Trends in medication treatment of hyperactive school children. In K. D. Gadow (Ed.), *Advances in learning and behavioral disabilities* (Vol. 3, pp. 125–149). Greenwich, CT: JAI Press.

Salvia, J. & Ysseldyke, J. E. (1981). *Assessment in special and remedial education.* Boston: Houghton-Mifflin.

Satterfield, J. H. J., Hoppe, C. M. & Schell, A. M. (1982). A prospective study of delinquency in 110 adolescent boys with attention deficit disorder and 88 normal adolescent boys. *American Journal of Psychiatry, 139,* 795–798.

Schaffer, D. (1985). Enuresis. In M. Rutter & L. Hersov (Eds.), *Child and adolescent psychiatry* (pp. 465–481). London: Blackwell Scientific.

Schenck, C. H., Bundlie, S. R., Patterson, A. L. & Mahowald, M. W. (1987). Rapid eye movement sleep behavior disorder: A treatable parasomnia affecting older adults. *Journal of the American Medical Association, 257,* 1786–1789.

Schroeder, S. R., Bicker, W. K. & Richmond, G. (1986). Primary and secondary prevention of self-injurious behavior: A lifelong problem. In K. D. Gadow (Ed.), *Advances in learning and behavioral disabilities* (Vol. 5, pp. 63–85). Greenwich, CT: JAI Press.

Schroeder, S. R., Schroeder, C. S., Smith, B. & Dalldorf, J. (1978). Prevalence of self-injurious behaviors in a large state facility for the retarded: A three-year follow-up study. *Journal of Autism and Childhood Schizophrenia, 8,* 261–269.

Segraves, R. T. (1989). Effects of psychotropic drugs on human erection and ejaculation. *Archives of General Psychiatry, 46,* 275–284.

Sepinwall, J. & Cook, L. (1978). Behavioral pharmacology of antianxiety drugs. In L. L. Iverson, S. D. Iverson & S. H. Snyder (Eds.), *Handbook of psychopharmacology* (pp. 345–393). New York: Plenum Press.

Shalev, A., Hermesh, H., & Munitz, H. (1989). Mortality from neuroleptic malignant syndrome. *Journal of Clinical Psychiatry, 50,* 18–25.

Shapiro, A. K. & Morris, L. A. (1978). The placebo effect in medical and psychological therapies. In S. L. Garfield & A. E. Bergin (Eds.), *Handbook of psychotherapy and behavioral change: An empirical analysis* (pp. 369–410). New York: John Wiley & Sons.

Shapiro, A. K., Shapiro, E., Young, J. G. & Feinberg, T. E. (1988). *Gilles de la Tourette syndrome.* New York: Raven Press.

Shapiro, E., Shapiro, A. K., Fulop, G., Hubbard, M., Mandeli, J., Nordlie, J. & Phillips, R. A. (1989). Controlled study of haloperidol, pimozide, and placebo for the treatent of Gilles de la Tourette's syndrome. *Archives of General Psychiatry, 46,* 722–730.

Shapiro, S., Hartz, S. C., Siskind, V., Mitchell, A. A., Slone, D., Rosenberg, L., Monson, R. R. & Heinonen, O. P. (1976). Anticonvulsants and parental epilepsy in the development of birth defects. *Lancet, 1,* 272–275.

Sheard, M. H. (1978). The effect of lithium and other ions on aggressive behavior. In L. Valzelli (Ed.), *Modern problems of pharmacopsychiatry* (Vol. 13, pp. 53–68). New York: Karger.

Sheehan, D. V. (1980). Panic attack and phobias. *New England Journal of Medicine, 307,* 156–158.

Sheehan, D. V., Ballenger, J. & Jacobsen, G. (1980). Treatment of endogenous anxiety with phobic, hysterical and hypochondrial symptoms. *Archives of General Psychiatry, 37,* 51–59.

Shen, W. W., Sata, L. S. & Hofstatter, L. (1984). Thioridazine and understanding sexual phases in both sexes. *Psychiatric Journal of the University of Ottawa, 9*, 187–190.

Simpson, G. M., & Angus, J. W. S. (1970). A rating scale for extrapyramidal side effects. *Acta Psychiatrica Scandinavica* (Suppl. 212), 11–19.

Singer, H. S., Gammon, K. & Quaskey, S. (1986). Haloperidol, fluphenizine and clonidine in Tourette syndrome: Controversies in treatment. *Pediatric Neuroscience, 12*, 71–74.

Singh, N. N. & Aman, M. G. (1981). Effects of thioridazine dosage on the behavior of several mentally retarded persons. *American Journal of Mental Deficiency, 85*, 580–587.

Singh, N. N. & Millichamp, C. J. (1985). Pharmacological treatment of self-injurious behavior in mentally retarded persons. *Journal of Autism and Developmental Disorders, 15*, 257–267.

Skolnick, P. & Paul, S. M. (1982). Benzodiazepine receptors in the central nervous system. *International Review of Neurobiology, 23*, 103–140.

Sleator, E. K. (1985). Measurement of compliance. *Psychopharmacology Bulletin, 21*, 1089–1093.

Sleator, E. K. & Sprague, R. L. (1978). Pediatric psychopharmacology. In W. G. Clark & J. del Guidice (Eds.), *Advances in learning and behavioral disabilities* (Vol. 1, pp. 341–364). Greenwich, CT: JAI Press.

Small, G. W. (1989). Tricyclic antidepressants for medically ill geriatric patients. *Journal of Clinical Psychiatry, 50*, 27–31.

Sneader, W. (1985).. *Drug discovery: The evolution of modern medicines.* New York: John Wiley & Sons.

Sprague, R. L. & Baxley, G. B. (1978). Drugs for behavior management, with comment on some legal aspects. In J. Wortis (Ed.), *Mental retardation and developmental disabilities* (Vol. 10, pp. 92–129). New York: Brunner/Mazel.

Sprague, R. L. Barnes, K. R. & Werry, J. S. (1970). Methylphenidate and thioridazine: Learning, reaction time, activity, and classroom behavior in emotionally disturbed children. *American Journal of Orthopsychiatry, 40*, 615–628.

Sprague, R. L., & Sleator, E. K. (1977). Methylphenidate in hyperkinetic children: Difference in dose effects on learning and social behavior. *Science, 198*, 1274–1276.

Sprague, R. L., & Werry, J. L. (1971). Methodology of psychopharmacological studies with the retarded. In N. R. Ellis (Ed.), *International review of research in mental retardation* (Vol. 5, pp. 147–219). New York: Academic Press.

Stimmel, G. L. & Escobar, J. I. (1986). Antidepressants in chronic pain: A review of efficacy. *Pharmacotherapy, 6*, 262–267.

Stores, G. (1985). Clinical and EEG evaluation of seizures and seizure-like disorders. *Journal of the American Academy of Child Psychiatry, 24*, 10–16.

Strober, M. & Carlson, G. A. (1982). Bipolar illness in adolescents with major depression. *Archives of General Psychiatry, 39*, 549–555.

Swinyard, E. A. (1982). Introduction. In D. M. Woodbury, J. K. Penry & C. E. Pippenger (Eds.), *Antiepileptic drugs* (pp. 1–10). New York: Raven Press.

Tapia, F. (1969). Haldol in the treatment of children with tics and stutterers—and an incidental finding. *Psychiatric Quarterly, 43*, 647–649.

Thorley, G. (1984). Review of follow-up and follow-back studies of childhood hyperactivity. *Psychological Bulletin, 96*, 116–132.

Tupin, J. P. & Schuller, A. B. (1978). Lithium and haloperidol incompatibility reviewed. *Psychiatry Journal of the University of Ottawa, 3*, 245–251.

van Praag, H. M. (1981). *Handbook of biological psychiatry: Drug treatment in psychiatry—psychotropic drugs.* New York: Dekker.

Van Scheyen, J. D. & Van Kamman, D. P. (1979). Clomipramine induced mania in unipolar depression. *Archives of General Psychiatry, 36*, 560–565.

Wagner, W., Johnson, S. B., Walker, D., Carter, R. & Wittner, J. (1982). A controlled comparison of two treatments for nocturnal enuresis. *Journal of Pediatrics, 101,* 302–307.

Wardell, D. W., Rubin, H. K. & Ross, R. T. (1958). The use of reserpine and chlorpromazine in disturbed mentally deficient patients. *American Journal of Mental Deficiency, 63,* 330–344.

Watt, D. C. (1975). Time to evaluate long-acting neuroleptics? *Psychological Medicine, 5,* 222–226.

Wehr, T. A., & Goodwin, F. K. (1979). Rapid cycling in manic-depressives induced by tricyclic antidepressants. *Archives of General Psychiatry, 36,* 555–559.

Wehr, T. A. & Goodwin, F. K. (1987). Can antidepressants cause mania and worsen the course of affective illness? *American Journal of Psychiatry, 144,* 1403–1411.

Weinstein, M. R. (1980). Lithium treatment of women during pregnancy and in the post-delivery period. In F. N. Johnson (Ed.), *Handbook of lithium therapy* (pp. 421–432). Lancaster, England: MTP Press.

Weiss, G. (1975). The natural history of hyperactivity in children and treatment with stimulant medication at different ages. *International Journal of Mental Health, 4,* 213–226.

Weiss, G., Kruger, E., Danielson, U. & Elman, M. (1975). Effects of long-term treatment of hyperactive children with methylphenidate. *Canadian Medical Association Journal, 112,* 159–165.

Weller, E. B., Weller, R. A. & Fristad, M. A. (1986). Lithium dosage guide for prepubertal children: A preliminary report. *Journal of the American Academy of Child Psychiatry, 25,* 92–95.

Wells, P. G. & Malcolm, M. T. (1971). Controlled trial of the treatment of 36 stutterers. *British Journal of Psychiatry, 119,* 603–604.

Werry, J. S. (1978). Measures in pediatric psychopharmacology. In J. S. Werry (Ed.), *Pediatric psychopharmacology: The use of behavior modifying drugs in children* (pp. 99–126). New York: Brunner/Mazel.

Werry, J. S. & Aman, M. G. (1975). Methylphenidate and haloperidol in children. *Archives of General Psychiatry, 32,* 790–795.

Werry, J. S., Aman, M. G. & Diamond, E. (1980). Imipramine and methylphenidate in hyperactive children. *Journal of Child Psychology and Psychiatry, 21,* 37–45.

Whalen, C. K. (1982). Hyperactivity, learning problems, and the attention deficit disorders. In T. H. Ollendick & M. Jersen (Eds.), *Handbook of child psychopathology* (pp. 151–199). New York: Plenum Press.

Whalen, C. K., Henker, B., Collins, E. B., Finck, D. & Dotemoto, S. (1979). A social ecology of hyperactive boys: Medication effects in systematically structured classroom environments. *Journal of Applied Behavior Analysis, 12,* 65–81.

White, L., Tursky, B. & Schwartz, G. E. (1985). *Placebo: Theory, research, and mechanisms.* New York: Guilford Press.

Williams, D. T. & Mostofsky, D. I. (1982). Psychogenic seizures in childhood and adolescence. In T. Riley & A. Roy (Eds.), *Pseudoseizures* (pp. 106–134). Baltimore: Williams & Wilkins.

Winsberg, B. G. & Yepes, L. E. (1978). Antipsychotics (major tranquilizers, neuroleptics). In J. S. Werry (Ed.), *Pediatric psychopharmacology: The use of behavior modifying drugs in children* (pp. 234–273). New York: Brunner/Mazel.

Woodbury, D. M., Penry, J. K. & Pippenger, C. E. (1982). *Antiepileptic drugs.* New York: Raven Press.

Wysocki, T., Fuqua, R. W., Davis, V. J. & Breuning, S. E. (1981). Effects of thioridazine (Mellaril) on titrating delayed matching-to-sample performance of mentally retarded adults. *American Journal of Mental Deficiency, 85,* 539–547.

Yassa, R., Camille, Y. & Belzile, L. (1987). Tardive dyskinesia in the course of antidepressant therapy: A prevalence study and review of the literature. *Journal of Clinical Psychopharmacology, 7,* 243–246.

Yepes, L., Balka, E., Winsberg, B. & Bialer, I. (1977). Amitriptyline and methylphenidate treatment of behaviorally disordered children. *Journal of Child Psychology and Psychiatry, 18,* 39–52.

Zimbardo, P. G. (1988). *Psychology and life.* Glenview, IL: Scott, Foresman.

Zimmerman, F. T. & Burgemeister, B. B. (1958). Action of methylphenidate (Ritalin) and reserpine in behavior disorders in children and adults. *American Journal of Psychiatry, 115,* 323–328.

Zimmermann, R. L. & Heistad, G. T. (1982). Studies of the long term efficacy of antipsychotic drugs in controlling the behavior of institutionalized retardates. *Journal of the American Academy of Child Psychiatry, 21,* 136–143.

Zubenko, G. S., Cohen, B. M. & Lipinski, J. F. (1987). Antidepressant-related akathisia. *Journal of Clinical Psychopharmacology, 7,* 254–257.

Selected Readings

CHAPTER 1

Gadow, K. D. (1986a). *Children on medication: Vol. 1. Hyperactivity, learning disabilities, and mental retardation*. San Diego: College-Hill Press.

Gadow, K. D. (1986b). *Children on medication: Vol. 2. Epilepsy, emotional disturbance, and adolescent disorders*. San Diego: College-Hill Press.

Gadow, K. D. & Poling, A. (1988). *Pharmacotherapy and mental retardation*. San Diego: College-Hill Press.

Gilman, A. G., Goodman, L. S., Rall, T. W. & Murad, F. (1985). *The pharmacological basis of therapeutics*. New York: Macmillan.

Klein, D. F., Gittelman, R., Quitkin, F. & Roifkin, A. (1980). *Diagnosis and drug treatment of psychiatric disorders: Adults and children*. Baltimore: Williams & Wilkins.

Leavitt, F. (1982). *Drugs and behavior*. Philadelphia: Saunders.

Werry, J. S. (1978). *Pediatric psychopharmacology: The use of behavior modifying drugs in children*. New York: Brunner/Mazel.

CHAPTER 2

Clark, W. G. & del Guidice, J. (1978). *Principles of psychopharmacology*. New York: Academic Press.

Gilman, A. G., Goodman, L. S., Rall, T. W. & Murad, F. (1985). *The pharmacological basis of therapeutics*. New York: Macmillan.

Goth, A. (1984). *Medical pharmacology*. St. Louis: Mosby.

Julien, R. M. (1985). *A primer of drug action*. New York: Freeman.

Lickey, M. E. & Gordon, B. (1983). *Drugs for mental illness*. New York: Freeman.

CHAPTER 3

Aman, M. G. & White, A. J. (1985). Measures of drug change in mental retardation. In K. D. Gadow (Ed.), *Advances in learning and behavioral disabilities* (Vol. 5, pp. 157–202). Greenwich, CT: JAI Press.

Crook, T., Ferris, S. & Bartus, R. (1983). *Assessment in geriatric psychopharmacology*. New Canaan, CT: Mark Powley Associates.

Gadow, K. D. & Poling, A. (1986). *Methodological issues in human psychopharmacology (Advances in learning and behavioral disabilities, Suppl. 1)* (pp. 41–84). Greenwich, CT: JAI Press.

Werry, J. S. (1978). Measures in pediatric psychopharmacology. In J. S. Werry (Ed.), *Pediatric psychopharmacology: The use of behavior modifying drugs in children* (pp. 99–126). New York: Brunner/Mazel.

White, L., Tursky, B. & Schwartz, G. E. (1985). *Placebo: Theory, research, and mechanisms*. New York: Guilford Press.

CHAPTER 4

Baldessarini, R. J. (1985). Drugs and the treatment of psychiatric disorders. In A. G. Gilman, L. S. Goodman, T. W. Rall & F. Murad (Eds.), *The pharmacological basis of therapeutics* (7th ed., pp. 387–445). New York: Macmillan.

Baldessarini, R. J., Cohen, B. M. & Teicher, M. H. (1988). Significance of neuroleptic dose and plasma level in the pharmacological treatment of psychoses. *Archives of General Psychiatry, 45,* 79–91.

Gadow, K. D. & Poling, A. (1988). *Pharmacotherapy and mental retardation*. Boston: Little, Brown.

Klein, D. F., Gittelman, R., Quitkin, F. & Rifkin, A. (1980). *Diagnosis and drug treatment of psychiatric disorders: Adults and children* (2nd ed.). Baltimore: Williams & Wilkins.

Lader, M. (1989). Clinical pharmacology of antipsychotic drugs. *Journal of International Medical Research, 17,* 1–16.

McEvoy, J. P. (1983). The clinical use of anticholinergic drugs as treatment for extrapyramidal side effects of neuroleptic drugs. *Journal of Clinical Psychopharmacology, 3,* 288–302.

Shapiro, A. K., Shapiro, E., Young, J. G. & Feinberg, T. E. (1988). *Gilles de la Tourette Syndrome* (2nd ed.). New York: Raven.

Winsberg, B. G. & Yepes, L. E. (1978). Antipsychotics (major tranquilizers, neuroleptics). In J. S. Werry (Ed.), *Pediatric psychopharmacology: The use of behavior modifying drugs in children* (pp. 234–273). New York: Brunner/Mazel.

CHAPTER 5

Lydiard, R. B., Roy-Byrne, P. P. & Ballenger, J. C. (1988). Recent advances in the psychopharmacological treatment of anxiety disorders. *Hospital and Community Psychiatry, 39,* 1157–1165.

McEvoy, G. K. (1988). *American hospital formulary service drug information 89*. New York: American Society of Hospital Pharmacists.

Meyer, K., Roth, T. & Dement, W. C. (1989). *Principles and practices of sleep medicine*. Philadelphia: W. B. Saunders.

Sepinwall, J. & Cook, L. (1978). Behavioral pharmacology of antianxiety drugs. In L. L. Iverson, S. D. Iverson & S. H. Snyder (Eds.), *Handbook of psychopharmacology* (pp. 345–393). New York: Plenum Press.

CHAPTER 6

Barkley, R. A. (1981). *Hyperactive children: A handbook for diagnosis and treatment.* New York: Guilford Press.
Gadow, K. D. (1986a). *Children on medication: Vol. I. Hyperactivity, learning disabilities, and mental retardation.* San Diego: College-Hill Press.
Pelham, W. E. & Murphy, A. (1986). Attention deficit and conduct disorders. In M. Hersen (Ed.), *Pharmacological and behavioral treatment: An integrative approach* (pp. 108–148). New York: John Wiley & Sons.
Ross, D. M. & Ross, S. A. (1982). *Hyperactivity: Current issues, research, and theory.* New York: John Wiley & Sons.

CHAPTER 7

Baldessarini, R. J. (1989). Current status of antidepressants: Clinical pharmacology and therapy. *Journal of Clinical Psychiatry, 50,* 117–126.
Blackwell, B. & Currah, J. (1973). The psychopharmacology of nocturnal enuresis. In I. Kalvin, R. C. MacKeith & S. R. Meadow (Eds.), *Bladder control and enuresis* (pp. 231–257). London: Heinemann.
Cantwell, D. P. & Carlson, G. A. (Eds.). (1983). *Affective disorders in childhood and adolescence: An update.* New York: Spectrum.
Johnson, F. N. (Ed.). (1980). *Handbook of lithium therapy.* Lancaster, England: MTP Press.
Klein, D. F., Gittelman, R., Quitkin, F. & Rifkin, A. (1980). *Diagnosis and drug treatment of psychiatric disorders: Adults and children* (2nd ed.). Baltimore: Williams & Wilkins.
Meltzer, H. Y. (Ed.), (1987). *Psychopharmacology: The third generation of progress.* New York: Raven Press.
Preskorn, S. H. (1989). Tricyclic antidepressants: The whys and hows of therapeutic drug monitoring. *Journal of Clinical Psychiatry, 50,* 34–42.

CHAPTER 8

Dreifuss, F. E. (1983). *Pediatric epileptology.* Littleton, MA: John Wright.
Gadow, K. D. (1986). *Children on medication: Vol. II. Epilepsy, emotional disturbance, and adolescent disorders.* San Diego: College-Hill Press.
Morselli, P. L., Pippenger, C. E. & Penry, J. E. (1983). *Antiepilepsy drug therapy in pediatrics.* New York: Raven Press.
Pietsch, S. (1977). *The person with epilepsy: Life style, needs, expectations.* Chicago: National Epilepsy League.
Rall, R. W. & Schliefer, L. S. (1985). Drugs effective in the therapy of the epilepsies. In A. G. Gilman, L. S. Goodman, T. W. Rall & F. Murad (Eds.), *The pharmacological basis of therapeutics* (pp. 446–472). New York: Macmillan.
Svoboda, W. B. (1979). *Learning about epilepsy.* Baltimore: University Park Press.
Woodbury, D. M., Penry, J. K. & Pippenger, C. E. (1982). *Antiepileptic drugs.* New York: Raven Press.

Author Index

Subject Index

About the Authors

Alan Poling received his Ph.D. in psychology in 1977. He is currently Professor of Psychology, Western Michigan University. His research interests are in behavioral pharmacology, learning processes, research methodology, and mental retardation, and he has written extensively in each of these areas. His books include *A Primer of Human Behavioral Pharmacology, Psychology: A Behavioral Overview, Pharmacotherapy and Mental Retardation,* and *Research Methods in Applied Behavior Analysis.*

Kenneth D. Gadow received his Ph.D. in special education from the University of Illinois in 1978. He is currently Professor of Special Education and Affiliate Professor of Child Psychiatry, State University of New York at Stony Brook. He is the author of *Children on Medication* (Vols. 1 & 2) and numerous journal articles, and the editor of the research annual, *Advances in Learning and Behavioral Disabilities.* His research interests are in pediatric psychopharmacology, hyperactivity, childhood aggression, and television violence.

James P. Cleary received his Ph.D. in psychology in 1982. He is currently Assistant Clinical Professor and Research Associate in the Department of Psychology, University of Minnesota. He is also Assistant Director of Education and Research Development for the Geriatric Research, Education and Clinical Center at the Veterans Administration Medical Center, Minneapolis. Dr. Cleary's primary research interests, and many of his publications, involve the behavioral effects of psychoactive drugs, particularly drugs of abuse. He conducts research on reducing analgesic drug self-administration, adjunct pharmacological treatment of pain, behavioral effects of opioid drugs, and pharmacological stimulation of eating.

Psychology Practitioner Guidebooks

Editors
Arnold P. Goldstein, Syracuse University
Leonard Krasner, Stanford University & SUNY at Stony Brook
Sol L. Garfield, Washington University in St. Louis

Elsie M. Pinkston & Nathan L. Linsk—CARE OF THE ELDERLY:
A Family Approach

Donald Meichenbaum—STRESS INOCULATION TRAINING

Sebastiano Santostefano—COGNITIVE CONTROL THERAPY WITH
CHILDREN AND ADOLESCENTS

Lillie Weiss, Melanie Katzman & Sharlene Wolchik—TREATING BULIMIA:
A Psychoeducational Approach

Edward B. Blanchard & Frank Andrasik—MANAGEMENT OF CHRONIC
HEADACHES: A Psychological Approach

Raymond G. Romanczyk—CLINICAL UTILIZATION OF
MICROCOMPUTER TECHNOLOGY

Philip H. Bornstein & Marcy T. Bornstein—MARITAL THERAPY:
A Behavioral-Communications Approach

Michael T. Nietzel & Ronald C. Dillehay—PSYCHOLOGICAL
CONSULTATION IN THE COURTROOM

Elizabeth B. Yost, Larry E. Beutler, M. Anne Corbishley & James R.
Allender—GROUP COGNITIVE THERAPY: A Treatment Approach for
Depressed Older Adults

Lillie Weiss—DREAM ANALYSIS IN PSYCHOTHERAPY

Edward A. Kirby & Liam K. Grimley—UNDERSTANDING AND
TREATING ATTENTION DEFICIT DISORDER

Jon Eisenson—LANGUAGE AND SPEECH DISORDERS IN CHILDREN

Eva L. Feindler & Randolph B. Ecton—ADOLESCENT ANGER
CONTROL: Cognitive-Behavioral Techniques

Michael C. Roberts—PEDIATRIC PSYCHOLOGY: Psychological
Interventions and Strategies for Pediatric Problems

Daniel S. Kirschenbaum, William G. Johnson & Peter M. Stalonas, Jr.—
TREATING CHILDHOOD AND ADOLESCENT OBESITY

W. Stewart Agras—EATING DISORDERS: Management of Obesity,
Bulimia and Anorexia Nervosa

Ian H. Gotlib & Catherine A. Colby—TREATMENT OF DEPRESSION:
An Interpersonal Systems Approach

Walter B. Pryzwansky & Robert N. Wendt—PSYCHOLOGY AS A
PROFESSION: Foundations of Practice

Cynthia D. Belar, William W. Deardorff & Karen E. Kelly—THE
PRACTICE OF CLINICAL HEALTH PSYCHOLOGY

Paul Karoly & Mark P. Jensen—MULTIMETHOD ASSESSMENT OF
CHRONIC PAIN

Margaret P. Korb, Jeffrey Gorrell & Vernon Van De Riet—GESTALT
THERAPY: Practice and Theory, Second Edition

Donald A. Williamson—ASSESSMENT OF EATING DISORDERS
Obesity, Anorexia, and Bulimia Nervosa

J. Kevin Thompson—BODY IMAGE DISTURBANCE:
Assessment and Treatment

William J. Fremouw, Maria de Perczel & Thomas E. Ellis—SUICIDE RISK:
Assessment and Response Guidelines

Arthur M. Horne & Thomas V. Sayger—TREATING CONDUCT AND
OPPOSITIONAL DEFIANT DISORDERS IN CHILDREN

Richard A. Dershimer—COUNSELING THE BEREAVED

Eldon Tunks & Anthony Bellissimo—BEHAVIORAL MEDICINE: Concepts
and Procedures

Alan Poling, Kenneth D. Gadow & James Cleary—DRUG THERAPY FOR
BEHAVIOR DISORDERS: An Introduction

Ira Daniel Turkat— THE PERSONALITY DISORDERS: A Psychological
Approach to Clinical Management

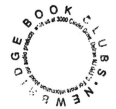